"Grant is a pioneer, enlightening and teaching us about neurodiversity-affirming practices for mental health professionals who provide play therapy for children. This book provides a clear and practical guide for structuring play therapy in meaningful ways to meet the needs of neurodivergent children."

Lynn Louise Wonders, *LPC, CPCS, RPT-S*™

"Robert Jason Grant contributes once again to the mental health field. In his new book, he offers structured and practical interventions grounded in the AutPlay® framework. Mental health therapists who want to increase their confidence and competence when working with neurodivergent children and adolescents will find this book extremely valuable."

Tony Lai, *MA, LPC, RPT-S*™

"*Play Interventions for Neurodivergent Children and Adolescents: Promoting Growth, Empowerment, and Affirming Practices* is a well-balanced and detailed book for anyone who is interested in providing fun and play based interventions for the neurodivergent client. Dr. Robert Jason Grant uses a concentrated lens to clearly show the importance of empathy and understanding when implementing play interventions with neurodivergent children. He details specific techniques to help with clients' social navigation, regulation, and feeling identification needs, as well as valuable information on the neurodiversity paradigm and ableist practices. This will be my new, go-to book; not only when working with my neurodivergent clients, but also when checking within to enhance my therapist abilities!"

Tracy Turner-Bumberry, *LPC, RPT-S*™

H01138824

Play Interventions for Neurodivergent Children and Adolescents

This revamped second edition provides several play interventions designed to address a variety of common mental health needs that neurodivergent children face, such as social navigation, regulation, relationship development, anxiety issues, identity struggles, and self-advocacy.

Completely reorganized and with the addition of several new chapters, the book begins with a thorough presentation of how and why structured interventions are used with neurodivergent children. Special focus is given to understanding neurodivergence, relationship and rapport building, therapy planning and goal setting, how to create a structured play intervention, the therapeutic powers of play, the role and level of involvement of the therapist, theory integration, avoiding ableist practices, and parent involvement. The second half of the book covers a wide selection of play therapy interventions for use with neurodivergent children and adolescents. The structured interventions focus on need areas related to social navigation, emotional expression, regulation, sensory processing, connection and relationship development, executive functioning, strengths, self-advocacy, and identity.

These structured play therapy interventions designed uniquely for neurodivergent children and adolescents will be valuable resources for any mental health professional working with neurodivergent youth.

Robert Jason Grant is a licensed professional counselor, national board-certified counselor, registered play therapist-supervisor, and a certified autism specialist based in Missouri, USA.

Play Interventions for Neurodivergent Children and Adolescents

Promoting Growth, Empowerment, and Affirming Practices

Second Edition

Robert Jason Grant

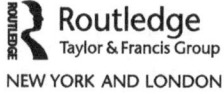
Routledge
Taylor & Francis Group

NEW YORK AND LONDON

Cover image © Getty Images

Second edition published 2024
by Routledge
605 Third Avenue, New York, NY 10158

and by Routledge
4 Park Square, Milton Park, Abingdon, Oxon, OX14 4RN

Routledge is an imprint of the Taylor & Francis Group, an informa business

© 2024 Robert Jason Grant

First edition published by Routledge 2016

Library of Congress Cataloging-in-Publication Data
Names: Grant, Robert Jason, 1971- author.
Title: Play interventions for neurodivergent children and adolescents: promoting growth, empowerment, and affirming practices /
Robert Jason Grant.
Other titles: Play-based interventions for autism spectrum disorder and other developmental disabilities
Description: Second edition. I New York, NY : Routledge, 2024. I
Revised edition of: Play-based interventions for autism spectrum disorder and other developmental disabilities / Robert Jason Grant. 2017. I
Identifiers: LCCN 2023024876 (print) I LCCN 2023024877
(ebook) I ISBN 9781032504841 (hbk) I ISBN 9781032504834 (pbk) I
ISBN 9781003398691 (ebk) Subjects: LCSH: Play therapy. I Autism in children--Treatment. I Autism spectrum disorders in children--Treatment. I
Neurodivergent children--Rehabilitation. I Neurodivergent youth--Rehabilitation. I Neurodivergent children--Counseling of. I Neurodivergent youth--Counseling of. Classification: LCC RJ505.P6 G735 2024 (print) I
LCC RJ505.P6 (ebook) I
DDC 618.92/85882--dc23/eng/20230822
LC record available at https://lccn.loc.gov/2023024876
LC ebook record available at https://lccn.loc.gov/2023024877

ISBN: 978-1-032-50484-1 (hbk)
ISBN: 978-1-032-50483-4 (pbk)
ISBN: 978-1-003-39869-1 (ebk)

DOI: 10.4324/9781003398691

Typeset in Sabon
by SPi Technologies India Pvt Ltd (Straive)

Contents

Foreword

Imagine walking into a space where the sounds were jarring, the colors discombobulating, the smells unfamiliar and strange, and there was not one comfortable space for you to find safety, quiet, and comfort. Now imagine that the majority of spaces you enter into throughout the day all feel like this, including the special place you go to where that nice person truly understands you, accepts you, advocates for you, and is trying to be there for you. Imagine how incongruent and confusing this would feel. The world of child and family therapy has been waiting for a book like *Play Interventions for Neurodivergent Children and Adolescents: Promoting Growth, Empowerment, and Affirming Practices* for a very long time.

It has long been assumed that neurodivergent children could not and would not appreciate or understand the value of play, let alone play therapy as a treatment approach. As our collective understanding of neurodiversity has grown, it is only natural that child and family therapists have been trying to improve their own play therapy practices, approach, and understanding of the clients we serve.

Understanding and making strides to shift our own adult ways of understanding the unique needs and abilities of our young clients is so very important. Play therapists have long heralded that play is the natural language of childhood. When we can go back to our roots, truly meet the child where the child is at developmentally, emotionally, mentally, socially, and physically, we can find the magic of what makes this work so very powerful and special. There is a natural human tendency to shy away from discomfort and in our polarized world, there is no better time than now to understand new information regarding neurodiversity and make the shifts needed in our play therapy approach and practice a safe space for all clients.

Dr. Grant's integrative play therapy approach in working with neurodivergent children and adolescents paves a pathway forward for new and seasoned clinicians to follow in order to eliminate unconscious bias, ableism, and non-affirming practices in the playroom. The book begins with a brief, but in-depth exploration of the neurodiversity paradigm and the how and why structured play therapy interventions are used with neurodivergent children. Readers will come away with new tools and resources for understanding neurodivergence, relationship and rapport building, therapy planning and goal setting, how to create a structured play intervention, the therapeutic powers of play, the role and level of involvement of the therapist, theory integration, avoiding ableist practices, and parent involvement.

The second half of the book contains a wide selection of play therapy interventions for use with neurodivergent children and adolescents. Chapters focus on structured interventions to improve social navigation, feeling identification, regulation, sensory processing, connection and relationship development, executive functioning, strengths, self-advocacy, and identity (self-worth). Special considerations for implementing structured interventions and an intervention tracking sheet are also included. Readers will come away with a clinical toolbox full of easy to implement play therapy interventions they can put into practice immediately.

Dr. Grant has been a trailblazer in the field of play therapy, championing the powers of play and neurodiversity alike. In his latest work, the interweaving of the beautiful tenets of play therapy and meeting the unique needs of our neurodivergent clients shines forth, as does his love and advocacy for access to play and play therapy for all children. May we all make a commitment to follow in these footsteps and begin advocating and practicing in a neurodiversity affirming manner.

Clair Mellenthin, LCSW, RPT-S™

Acknowledgments

I want to thank Routledge and my editor who allowed a second edition of this book so I could fully and freely create resources that are neurodiversity affirming. It has been a satisfying experience to update play therapy interventions and create new ones that truly honor neurodivergence while helping children address their mental health needs.

I am especially thankful for those who contributed interventions to this book. Thank you for sharing your energy and creativity. Each shared intervention provides a valuable contribution to this book. Thank you to those who provided reviews and those who have supported this project and encouraged me along the way.

Thank you to the play therapy and neurodivergent communities – you are always inspiring and always supportive, and that is greatly appreciated.

1 The Neurodiversity Paradigm and Ableist Practices

The Neurodiversity Paradigm

This book is not intended to provide a thorough or in-depth presentation of the neurodiversity paradigm and neurodivergence. The following is presented to help practitioners have a better understanding of neurodivergence as it relates to implementing structured play interventions. A suggested reading list is offered in the Appendix for those who wish to increase their knowledge about neurodivergence.

A paradigm is often defined as a distinct set of concepts or thought patterns, including theories, and research methods for what constitute legitimate contributions to a field. Simply put, it is a standard or set of ideas or way of looking at something. The neurodiversity paradigm is indeed a somewhat 'new' way of looking at the existence of neurodiversity within humans. In 1998, Autistic sociologist Judy Singer and journalist Harvey Blume coined the word neurodiversity as the range of natural diversity that exists in human neurodevelopment. This began a more thoughtful collective framework for Autistic and neurodivergent advocacy (Pellicano and Houting, 2021).

The neurodiversity paradigm takes the basic concept of neurodiversity and proposes that some brains are neurotypical (broadly conforming to a societal standard of 'normal'), and some brains are neurodivergent (that is, diverging from the societal standard, typically developing norm). The neurodiversity paradigm also proposes that divergent brains should exist alongside neurotypical brains, without judgement. Neurodivergent individuals are not 'disordered' (a subjective judgement) because of their neurodivergence. The paradigm proposes that typically developing brains are no more 'right' or 'desirable' than divergent brains (Heyworth, 2021; Walker, 2021).

The neurodiversity paradigm doesn't presume to judge which neurodivergences (even within the typically developing population) are valuable and which are not. It also doesn't presume to categorize neurodivergences into 'healthy' or 'deviant' differences. The neurodiversity paradigm doesn't deny the challenges associated with being neurodivergent. Although it does acknowledge that many such challenges would be lessened if appropriate accommodations were put in place through implementing the principles of affirming neurodivergence and eliminating ableist practices (Heyworth, 2021).

DOI: 10.4324/9781003398691-1

Pellicano and Houting (2021) stated that the neurodiversity paradigm promotes neurodivergent acceptance, urging people to embrace neurodivergence as an inherent and integral part of a person's identity and experience of the world. The potential value of this acceptance mind-set to neurodivergence is further supported by recent research indicating that greater neurodivergent identity understanding and acceptance are associated with better mental health.

Neurodivergence

Neurodivergence is the term for people whose brains function differently in one or more ways than is considered standard or typical. Neurodivergence refers to any structured, consistent way that brains work differently for a group of people than they do for the majority of others. It is estimated that over 1.2 billion people identify as neurodivergent (Grant, 2023).

A neurodivergent child is in contrast to a neurotypical child. The basic definition of a neurodivergent person is anyone whose brain processing, navigating, learning, etc. does not 'fit' the societal standard of what is considered typical or normal. Arguably the quickest way to identify a neurodivergent child would be through diagnoses such as Autistic, ADHD, learning differences, sensory differences, gifted, etc.; although a child does not have to have a diagnosis to be neurodivergent.

Neurodivergence is most definitely considered an identity (a type of diversity) and neurodiversity affirming is directly related to how a neurodivergent child is treated, accepted, and valued in systems and society as a whole. Will the neurodivergent child's different ways of navigating be accepted and appreciated or will they be devalued? This is the difference between being affirming versus not affirming (which often mirrors ableist practices).

Being Neurodiversity Affirming

Grant (2022) proposed that being neurodiversity affirming is a belief and commitment in approach, which means valuing and respecting the different ways a neurodivergent client may process, feel, respond, communicate, and play. It means allowing the child to be themself and not trying to change them to fit a neurotypical standard. Further, it means giving the client a voice in the decision-making process regarding their therapy. Thus, neurodiversity affirming is the act of valuing neurodiversity and affirming a child's neurotype.

Neurodiversity affirming is a commitment to putting forth relationship, interactions, processes, and approaches that value and uplift the child's neurotype, respecting their neurodivergence. The neurodiversity affirming practitioner will take care to empower the neurodivergent child as opposed to trying to make them look neurotypical. The child's neurodivergence will be accepted as opposed to pathologized. For the practitioner, it means fully recognizing and accepting the child's neurodivergence. It means acknowledging the child's different neuro system which includes their strengths. It also means providing the child with the support and accommodations needed and doing this in a way that empowers and respects the child (Grant, 2022).

Ableism

Understanding neurodiversity, neurodivergence, and being neurodiversity affirming must include a thorough awareness of ableism. The term 'ableism' is often defined as discrimination and social prejudice against people with disabilities or who are perceived to have disabilities (including neurodivergent individuals). Ableism characterizes people as defined by their disabilities and as inferior to the non-disabled. On this basis, people are assigned or denied certain perceived abilities, skills, or character orientations. Ableism can take the form of ideas and assumptions, stereotypes, attitudes and practices, physical barriers in the environment, or larger scale oppression (Grant, 2023).

Ableism and ableist practices can manifest (and often do) in any system or setting including mental health care and play therapy. Reeve (2000) identified ableism in therapy practice where practitioners employ a predominantly medical model of disability that risks discounting alternative relational understandings. In therapy, disability and neurodivergence are constructed in relation to the normal. Disability and/or neurodivergence are always understood as a problematic deviation from the normal, as an imperfection when judged against what is considered normative (neurotypical). There is a risk of needing to 'fix' or 'cure' something that is a part of how the person identifies. This can manifest through the practitioner's attitude, approach, and microaggressions communicated in structured play interventions and therapy goals.

Practitioners who work with neurodivergent children and adolescents should strive to become thoroughly educated about the many aspects related to the neurodiversity paradigm before implementing play interventions or any therapies with this population. Practitioners are encouraged to learn more about neurodivergence from neurodivergent individuals, understand the common mental health needs of children, be informed about helpful and affirming therapy approaches, and understand how to provide empowerment, identity awareness, advocacy, and healthy self-worth. Proper education about neurodivergence will enhance and elevate the implementation of play interventions for greater success.

For editing purposes, this book will often refer to neurodivergence and neurodivergent children in general instead of discussing various neurominorities. The play interventions in this book address the commonly shared mental health needs and struggles that can accompany most neurodivergent children and adolescents. These need areas include but are not limited to social navigation, feelings identification and expression, sensory needs, regulation needs, executive function needs, connection and relationship development, strengths development, identity and self-worth, and advocacy. Each neurominority will have specific characteristics that make them different from other neurominorities, and each neurodivergent child will have their individual needs and strengths. Practitioners are encouraged to increase their awareness of the specific child they are working with and understand that child's neurodivergent spectrum of presentation.

References

Grant, R. J. (2022). *Understanding sensory differences: A neurodiversity affirming guidebook for children and teens.* AutPlay Publishing.

Grant, R. J. (2023). *The AutPlay therapy handbook: An integrative family play therapy with neurodivergent children.* Routledge.

Heyworth, M. (2021). Introduction to Autism, Part 5: Neurodiversity (What is it and why do we care?). *Reframing Autism.* https://reframingautism.org.au/introduction-to-autism-part-5-neurodiversity-what-is-it-and-why-do-we-care/

Pellicano, E., & Houting, J. D. (2021). Annual Research Review: Shifting from 'normal science' to neurodiversity in autism science. *The Journal of Child Psychology and Psychiatry, 63*(4), 381–396.

Reeve, D. (2000). Oppression within the counselling room. *Disability & Society, 15*(4), 669–682.

Walker, N. (2021). *Neuroqueer heresies: Notes on the neurodiversity paradigm, autistic empowerment, and postnormal possibilities.* Autonomous Press.

2 Relationship Development and Rapport Building

Relationship Development

As with any therapeutic approach, it is essential that relationship building be a central focus. Practitioners should spend time in the beginning of therapy and throughout the totality of therapy building the relationship with children, adolescents, and the parents they are working with. Implementing structured play interventions, no matter how great the intervention, will be much less effective without the proper relationship and rapport between the practitioner and the child. Essentially, it is the relationship that gives the intervention value. Engaging with interventions in the right frame of mind will yield better results.

The purpose of a therapeutic relationship is to assist the child and family in therapy to change their life for the better. Such a relationship is essential, as it is oftentimes the first setting in which the person receiving therapy explores intimate thoughts, beliefs, and emotions regarding the issue(s) in question. As such, it is very important that practitioners provide a safe, open, and non-judgmental atmosphere where the child can be at ease. Trust, acceptance, and congruence are major components of a good therapeutic relationship. Practitioners are encouraged to show empathy and genuineness (Madeson, 2021).

Child-centered play therapy (CCPT) forms the foundation for building the relationship with the child. Landreth (1991) describes CCPT as an encompassing philosophy for living one's life in relationship with children. It is not a reference of techniques that are implemented in the playroom. It is a way of being based on a deep commitment to certain beliefs about children and their innate capacity for growth. It is a complete therapeutic process and not just the application of a few rapport-building techniques. It is based on the belief in the capacity and resiliency of children.

Landreth (2001) stated that the relationship is key to the growth and success of the therapeutic encounter. The most significant resource the practitioner brings to the relationship is the dimension of self. Landreth furthered by revising and expanding the eight personality qualities of the play therapist (originally created by Virginia Axline) that serve as the guide for fostering the therapeutic relationship. The practitioner working with neurodivergent

DOI: 10.4324/9781003398691-2

children can find this guide useful in implementing some or all parts in their relationship development goals:

1. The therapist is genuinely interested in the child and develops a warm, caring relationship.
2. The therapist experiences unqualified acceptance of the child and does not wish that the child was different in some way.
3. The therapist creates a feeling of safety and permissiveness in the relationship so that the child feels free to explore and express self completely.
4. The therapist is always sensitive to the child's feelings and gently reflects those feelings in such a manner that the child develops self-understanding.
5. The therapist believes deeply in the child's capacity to act responsibly, unwaveringly respects the child's ability to solve personal problems, and allows the child to do so.
6. The therapist trusts the child's inner direction, allows the child to lead in all areas of the relationship, and resists any urge to direct the child's play or conversation.
7. The therapist appreciates the gradual nature of the therapeutic process and does not attempt to hurry the process.
8. The therapist establishes only those therapeutic limits that help the child accept personal and appropriate relationship responsibility

(pp. 24–28)

In AutPlay therapy (Grant, 2023), relationship development begins with the initial phone call or email and appointment scheduling. Once an appointment is made, the parents are sent a social story that describes coming to see the play therapist and participating in play therapy. This story describes the process and provides pictures of the spaces the child may be in and pictures of the practitioner. The parents are instructed to read the story three times a day with their child, starting around four to five days prior to the appointment.

When a child arrives for their first appointment, they already have a familiarity with the space and the practitioner. Relationship development has begun before the practitioner and child meet in person. In AutPlay therapy protocol, the first four sessions focus on creating comfort for the child. The sessions are sensitive to the anxiety and dysregulation that may be present for the child coming into a new place and being with a new person. The focus is on helping the child feel safe in the play space and with the practitioner. If structured play interventions are implemented, they do not start until session five at the earliest.

Relationship development with many neurodivergent children happens in the context of presence, felt acceptance, and safety. Neurodivergent children may not 'show' relationship development to the practitioner in the way a neurotypical child might. This does not mean relationship development has not occurred for the neurodivergent child. The practitioner should be mindful to not make judgments about how the neurodivergent child experiences relationship. The following guides present ideas for practitioners in developing relationship with neurodivergent children:

1. Lead with creating safety, comfort, and acceptance with the child. Strive to understand how these concepts are felt by the child and provide that presence.
2. Do not place judgment on the child and/or the parents. Appreciate that neurodivergent children will present and navigate in ways that are different from neurotypical children. Show this appreciation to the child.
3. Do not over focus on or mislabel a child's behavior. Accept the child and the child's behavior where they are at with an understanding that dysregulated states often produce behavior and require empathic responding from the practitioner.
4. Provide unconditional positive regard to the child and parents.
5. Provide attunement, reflective responding, tracking, and active listing skills. These CCPT skills communicate 'I see you', 'I accept you', 'I am here with you'.
6. Allow and provide opportunities for the child to show you their play preferences and interests. Value their way of playing and interests; join them in these spaces, and do not discredit their play.
7. Maintain relationship development as an active process throughout the duration of therapy.

Burke (2021) described four lessons for developing the therapeutic relationship. The following are presented and adapted for working with neurodivergent children and adolescents.

Do not infantilize clients. Assume competence when interacting with children. This is especially important with neurodivergent children who may have high support needs.

Allow clients to be experts on their own lives. The goal is to help clients make meaning of their life, not ascribe our meaning to their life. Allow and value the child's voice to be heard. Appreciate that they have an awareness about themselves and how they enjoy life. It is not about turning them into the expression of what the practitioner thinks someone's life should look like.

Allow clients to feel that they matter. One of the most effective ways to do this is simply to ask children, 'Are you getting what you need?' 'Do you think this helps you?' Most children, especially neurodivergent children, are used to adults talking over them and for them. Communicating to children that they matter means helping them understand that their thoughts, feelings, and expressions are wanted and respected.

Seek out exceptional supervision. Consult with, gain supervision services, or simply learn from neurodivergent adults and other neurodivergent practitioners. This will greatly increase the practitioner's knowledge about neurodivergence and create better relationship processes between the practitioner and the child.

Regardless of the intervention being used, the practitioner/child relationship is central to the child's realization of therapy goals. The rapport that develops between the practitioner and child forms the foundation for therapeutic success. In building a therapeutic alliance, the practitioner must create an atmosphere of safety in which the child is made to feel accepted, understood, and respected (Lowenstein, 1999). Play-based interventions lend themselves to creating a very structured and directive session with a child or adolescent. The directive element of play interventions should not displace the importance for the practitioner and the child to develop a good rapport and relationship.

References

Burke, A. M. (2021). Four lessons in building therapeutic relationships. *Counseling Today.* https://ct.counseling.org/2021/11/four-lessons-in-building-therapeutic-relationships/

Grant, R. J. (2023). *The AutPlay therapy handbook: Integrative family play therapy with neurodivergent children.* Routledge.

Landreth, G. L. (1991). *Play therapy: The art of the relationship.* Psychology Press.

Landreth, G. L. (2001). *Innovations in play therapy: Issues, process, and special populations.* Routledge.

Lowenstein, L. (1999). *Creative interventions for troubled children & youth.* Highnell Book Printing.

Madeson, M. (2021). Therapeutic relationships in counseling: 4 phases explained. *Positive Psychology.* https://positivepsychology.com/therapeutic-relationship-phases/

3 Therapy Planning and Goal Setting

Therapy Planning

The American Psychological Association (2023) described mental health as an essential part of children's overall health. It has a complex interactive relationship with their physical health and their ability to succeed in school, at work, and in society. Both physical and mental health affect how the child thinks, feels, and acts on the inside and outside. Mental health is important throughout childhood, from prenatal considerations through transitions to adulthood.

It is important for practitioners to understand psychological theories and have a theoretical framework from which to work when providing mental health therapy, and especially when implementing structured interventions to address therapy goals (Cavett, 2010). Structured play interventions should always be grounded in a theoretical approach. The interventions in this book align with the AutPlay therapy protocol for structured play interventions to address the mental health needs of neurodivergent children and adolescents. AutPlay is an integrative family play therapy framework specifically designed to address the mental health needs of neurodivergent children. The AutPlay framework is an integration of seminal play therapy theories including child-centered play therapy, cognitive behavioral play therapy, filial therapy, Gestalt play therapy, and Theraplay® (Grant, 2017; Grant, 2023).

Structured play interventions should be specifically chosen to address mental health needs that an individual child or adolescent is struggling with. Interventions should be a component of the child's therapy plan and align with established therapy goals. Practitioners should be able to communicate why interventions are chosen for a specific child, how the intervention will help address the child's identified needs, how the intervention is a 'best fit' for the child, and how the intervention addresses the child's therapy goals. Practitioners should also implement evaluation procedures to assess whether the chosen play interventions are helping the child address targeted needs and that the child is making progress toward their established therapy goals.

When a neurodivergent child or adolescent is entering therapy, the first affirming step that the practitioner should do is ask, 'What are the mental health

DOI: 10.4324/9781003398691-3

needs?' 'Why is the neurodivergent child coming to therapy?' A neurodivergent child does not need any therapy simply because they are neurodivergent. There are plenty of Autistic and other neurodivergent children, adolescents, and adults who are not in any therapy and do not need any. The practitioner will begin the process of understanding what the mental health needs of the child are and whether the therapy is an appropriate support for the child's life.

Neurodivergent children, like any other children, can have mental health needs which require therapy to help support and/or resolve. Some common needs (therapy goals) for children in general (which includes neurodivergent children) can be struggling with a parent's divorce, dealing with grief and loss, parent/child relationship strain, life transitions, child abuse and neglect, trauma issues, and attachment issues. Some needs that may be more signifi-cant for neurodivergent children include feeling identification and expression (alexithymia), system regulation, social navigation needs (bullying, safety awareness, the social model of disability), relationship and connection, sensory needs, executive functioning needs, anxiety and depression, low self-worth, identity awareness needs, advocacy support, as well as trauma-related issues.

Therapy Planning and Play Interventions

Regardless of the mental health needs identified and being addressed through play therapy, the practitioner should review the following considerations for therapy goal planning and structured play interventions with neurodivergent children:

A *careful consideration of intersectionality.* Culture, ethnicity, and lan-guage influence the behavior of children in numerous ways, and as a result, affect the methods of mental health promotion and the preven-tion and therapy of mental health disorders (American Psychological Association, 2023). Therapy planning should consider diversity needs, as noted disparities exist for children living in low-income communities, ethnic minority children, those defined by gender identity and sexual orientation, immigration status, physical, developmental, and intellec-tual disabilities, and chronic medical conditions.

Interventions should address therapy goals. Structured play interventions are not random and without intent. They should be chosen and imple-mented in part, based on the practitioner's understanding that the inter-vention will help address identified therapy goals. A practical way to think about intervention implementation is to consider if someone were to observe an intervention being implemented, could the practitioner respond with a clear explanation of how it addressed therapy goals? This is what the practitioner is striving for when selecting and imple-menting play interventions.

Focus on one to two goals at a time. It is possible that a neurodivergent child will present for therapy with multiple identified therapy goals. The practitioner should not try to address all therapy goals at once. This could become overwhelming for both the practitioner and the child. Instead, one or two (no more than two) goals should be selected based on what seems to be priority needs. Once these goals have been achieved, one or two more goals can then be addressed. This can continue until all original goals have been addressed. Occasionally goals can be layered and somewhat mesh together. Likewise, some structured play interventions are designed to address more than one need area. This can be helpful, but the practitioners should caution that they have a clear view of what, how, and why things are happening in therapy, and where progress currently presents and what the movement forward looks like.

Goal progression will vary with neurodivergent children. Neurodivergent children and adolescents present on a spectrum of presentation. This means that each child will have different strengths and needs, each child will have their own unique spectrum of presentation. Some children will have more support needs, and some will have less. Because of this diversity (and other factors such as the level of parent involvement), progression with therapy goals will vary from child to child. Neuronormative is not synonymous with neurodivergent. The practitioner should not expect every neurodivergent child to respond positively to the same play interventions and progress though therapy goals at the same rate.

Implement an evaluation process. Because it is impossible to predict how long a neurodivergent child will participate in play therapy, the practitioner will want to devise an evaluation process to ensure progress is being made toward therapy goals. The evaluation can be done many ways but should be implemented periodically (every three to six months of therapy), involve the parents and child (if applicable), and have some type of evaluative component. The evaluative component could be a formal pre and post inventory, a question-and-answer session with the parents and child, or another method the practitioner implements. The goal is to thoroughly assess if progress has been made toward therapy goals. Progress does not have to move at a certain speed or amount (progression for the neurodivergent child may be very different than a neurotypical adult's view) but there should be recognized progress.

Developing a therapy plan and therapy goals is essential as neurodivergent children do not need to be in therapy if there are no therapy needs. It is a large responsibility of the practitioner to identify accurate (real) mental health therapy goals. If using structured play interventions, the practitioner must also understand how the interventions align with the therapy goals to meet the mental health needs of the neurodivergent child.

References

American Psychological Association (2023). Children's mental health. https://www.apa.org/topics/children/mental-health

Cavett, A. (2010). *Structured play-based interventions for engaging children and adolescents in therapy*. Infinity Publishing.

Grant, R. J. (2017). *AutPlay therapy for children and adolescents on the autism spectrum: A behavioral play-based approach*. Routledge.

Grant, R. J. (2023). *The AutPlay therapy handbook: Integrative family play therapy with neurodivergent children*. Routledge.

4   Creating Structured Play Interventions

Structured Play Interventions

Implementing structured play therapy interventions is based on the idea that the practitioner introduces interventions which they believe would be helpful for the child to complete to address therapy goals (Grant, 2017). In play therapy, this would mostly be done working from a directive theory or approach, which contrasts with a non-directive theory or approach which would not introduce structured interventions.

The concept is not new to the play therapy field. Jones et al. (2003) provided guidelines for planning and selecting toys and materials that are based on the model of structured play therapy. Hambidge (1955) developed a structured play therapy method which was implemented only after a relationship had already been established through nondirective play therapy. His method promoted a slow start, using fewer threatening toys and materials to recreate upsetting events, and then using the play to recover from the events (Leggett and Boswell, 2017).

Leggett and Boswell (2017) conceptualized three stages of a structured play therapy model which included opening, working through, and termination:

> 'These stages begin with a low intensity before increasing that intensity to its highest point during the working-through stage and then decreasing it as the termination stage approaches. The directive or structured activities and techniques are selected to create the desired level of intensity for each session. These levels are defined as (a) evoke anxiety, (b) challenge to self-disclose, (c) increase awareness, (d) focus on feelings, (e) focus on the here and now, and (f) focus on the threatening issues (Jones et al., 2003)'.
>
> (p. 3)

This book presents a preferred guide regarding the structured play interventions listed, indicating what level is appropriate for each intervention. The levels are listed as child, adolescent, or both child and adolescent. Most of the interventions in this book could be used for children ages 3 to 18 if the content (instructions and expectations) were adjusted adequately to reflect the child's age. Also, the child's cognitive understanding should be considered as

DOI: 10.4324/9781003398691-4

some neurodivergent children may present with development that is not equal to their chronological age.

Practitioners should not be hesitant about trying any of the interventions listed in this book with any of the children and adolescents they work with. It will be clear if an intervention is too advanced for the child's chronological or developmental age, and likewise, it will be clear if the intervention is too basic. If a practitioner realizes the intervention is too advanced or too basic, then adjustments can be made to fit the intervention to what is appropriate for the child.

Interventions in this book provide the primary therapy needs that the intervention addresses. This is a guide, as most of the interventions have multiple benefits, some that may not be indicated. Many of the interventions in the book have a social navigation and connection element – these needs can be addressed through a variety of the interventions, even though they may not be specifically listed in those two sections of the book. Also provided are the materials needed and the modality of individual, family, and/or group work. Again, even though recommendations are provided, many of these interventions can be used in any of these modalities.

Considerations for Creating Interventions

Practitioners wanting to create their own play interventions or implement interventions that they have learned from another source are encouraged to utilize the Create Your Own Intervention worksheet located in the Appendix section of this book. Some additional constructs for successful implementation with neurodivergent children are provided: *Simple in Instruction*: Neurodivergent children are less likely to focus on and engage in an intervention if the instructions are too long, complicated, or involve too many steps to complete the intervention. For interventions that may have multiple steps, it is helpful to present each step one at time, and allow the child to complete a step before presenting the next step. Ideally, the intervention can be easily adjusted from simple to more complex to match the child's needs.

Low Prop Based

Neurodivergent children may become distracted or over stimulated with too many toys, props, and expressive art materials around them or available to them. Keeping props simple and focused on the intervention being presented will aid in helping the child maintain focus and engagement, and ultimately aid in successful completion of the intervention. Practitioners may even want to present the intervention in an environment that is somewhat sterile and low on possible distractions.

Easily Implemented Across Various Environments

Many different practitioners in various settings work with neurodivergent children and adolescents. The interventions are ideally designed to transfer across many environments such as a play therapy room, a school counselor's office, an in-home setting, etc. Often, parents are involved in the therapy process, thus, interventions should also be easily implemented by parents in the home setting.

Targeted Toward Specific Therapy Needs

Interventions should be grounded in a theoretical base and chosen for a child or adolescent specifically to address identified therapy needs and goals. Interventions should align with and be part of the greater therapy plan that has been conceptualized for the individual child or adolescent and family.

Align With the Child's Play Preferences and Interests

Implementing interventions that align with the child's play preferences and their special interests will yield greater engagement and commitment to the intervention. This will ultimately produce better outcomes for the intervention, helping to address therapy goals.

Be More Playful Than Educational

Play is the natural language of all children and play holds the therapeutic components. As interventions are implemented, the practitioner should strive to be playful and make the interventions about the play and not a teaching/educational lesson.

Be Flexible and Allow for In The Moment Adjustments

The practitioner should be prepared for anything when implementing a play intervention. Possibly the child will not like it, maybe there will be a sensory or trauma trigger. While every effort should be made to ensure the intervention is a good fit for the child, there is still an unknown element. The practitioner will want to be flexible and able to adapt quickly and shift whatever is necessary in the moment.

Incorporate Multiple Points of Intervention

Ideally, interventions should incorporate more than one element (social, emotional regulation, anxiety reduction, sensory processing, connection, etc.). This provides the opportunity to address multiple therapy needs through the implementation of one intervention.

Avoid Teaching or Promoting Masking

Masking is defined as hiding and/or denying one's neurodivergent self or characteristics to be accepted and avoid shaming and rejection. It is often implemented as a survival response. Over time, it can produce depression, anxiety, low self-worth, and other mental health needs. Play interventions, especially those involving social navigation goals, must be scrutinized to avoid promoting masking.

AutPlay Therapy
NEURODIVERSITY-AFFIRMING PLAY INTERVENTION
Five Step Filtering Process

Pre-contemplation	Evaluation	Evaluation	Adjustment	Implementation
1	**2**	**3**	**4**	**5**
PLAY INTERVENTION	APPLICABLE FOR THERAPY GOALS	APPLICABLE TO THE CHILD	NEURODIVERSITY AFFIRMING	READY TO GO
Discovery, learning, or awareness of a new play therapy intervention.	Does the intervention address the child's therapy needs? In what way?	Does the intervention fit the child's needs, play preferences, and neurodivergent presentation?	Does the intervention promote masking or devaluing identity? Does it need adjusting in any way?	It's time to implement the intervention with the child.

Figure 4.1 The AutPlay therapy filtering process for neurodiversity affirming play therapy interventions.

Robert Jason Grant (2023)

Be Filtered to Ensure They Are Affirming

Play interventions come from many different sources. Many play interventions are not created specifically for or with consideration of neurodivergent children. The practitioner will need to evaluate any intervention they discover to make sure it is affirming and does not contain ableist concepts. Figure 4.1 provides a visual representation of the AutPlay therapy filtering process to ensure interventions are affirming.

Structured play interventions can be implemented in a single session and contained within that session experience, or they can be ongoing interventions that are repeated from session to session. Further, some interventions can be implemented as a pre and post measure to show progress and growth toward therapy goals. The utilization and implementation of play interventions will be constructed by the practitioner and with an understanding of how, when, and why.

References

Grant, R. J. (2017). *Play-based interventions for autism spectrum disorder and other developmental disabilities.* Routledge.

Hambidge, G. (1955). *Structured play therapy. American handbook for building the play therapy relationship.* Jason Aronson.

Jones, K. D., Casado, M., & Robinson, E. H. (2003). Structured play therapy: A model for choosing topics and activities. *International Journal of Play Therapy, 12*, 31–37.

Leggett, E. S., & Boswell, J. N. (2017). *Directive play therapy: Theories and techniques.* Springer Publishing Company.

5 Play Therapy and the Therapeutic Powers of Play

Play Therapy

Play therapy can best be thought of as an umbrella term, as there are currently several play therapy theories and approaches that exist (Crenshaw et al., 2015). Play therapy approaches range from being nondirective to directive in terms of the therapist's involvement in the process with their clients. Some theories and approaches of play therapy rely heavily on the use of toys and props, while other theories use toys minimally. Most play therapy approaches involve some use of toys, props, art, music, movement, or games as an avenue to help clients achieve their therapeutic goals. The Association for Play Therapy (2023) defines play therapy as the systematic use of a theoretical model to establish an interpersonal process wherein trained play therapists use the therapeutic powers of play to help clients prevent or resolve psychosocial difficulties and achieve optimal growth and development.

Currently, the Association for Play Therapy recognizes ten seminal and/or historically significant play therapy theories and approaches. The list includes Adlerian, child-centered, cognitive-behavioral, developmental (Viola Brody), ecosystemic, filial, Gestalt, Jungian, object-relations, and Theraplay. Beyond these ten recognized, there exist several established and emerging play therapy theories, approaches, and modalities such as sand tray therapy, family play therapy, experiential play therapy, expressive play therapy, relationship play therapy, first play, AutPlay therapy, digital play therapy, TraumaPlay, solution focused play therapy, synergetic play therapy, and animal-assisted play therapy – to name a few.

Play is considered the natural language of all children (Landreth, 1991). The benefits of children engaging in play include cognitive development (learning, thinking, and planning, etc.), social navigation (practicing social interaction, roles, and routines), language (communication stye, advocacy, turn taking, etc.), problem solving (negotiation, asking for help, solving difficulties, etc.), and emotional development (managing feelings, understanding others, empathy, etc.). Through play expression opportunities, children are more likely to be satisfied with peer relationships, and play is a key learning tool through which children can develop social navigation, regulation, core learning skills, and expression. Play also provides opportunities for children

DOI: 10.4324/9781003398691-5

to practice troubling events, situations, and routines in a safe place, with no pressure to 'get it right' (Phillips and Beavan, 2010).

Play therapy has not always been considered a viable approach for working with Autistic and other neurodivergent children. In fact, using any type of play approach to working with Autistic and other neurodivergent children was considered ineffective and a waste of time. The leading, misinformed, and often harmful belief that neurodivergent children did not play, did not understand play, and play held no therapeutic value for them, permeated many neurodivergent-focused 'treatments' for decades. Ableist thinking and processes guided many neurodivergent-related therapies as these children were often viewed as the equivalent of an animal that required training (Grant, 2023).

Sherratt and Peter (2002) suggested that play interventions and experiences are extremely important to neurodivergent children. They state that simultaneously activating the areas of the brain associated with emotions and generative thought while explicitly allowing neurodivergent children to play will lead to success. Further, Thornton and Cox (2005) conducted individual play sessions with Autistic children specifically to address behavior concerns. They incorporated play interventions which included relationship development, executive functioning, turn taking, enjoyment, and structure. Their research found that play interventions did impact on the child's behavior with a reduction in need areas following the structured play interventions.

Cross (2010) stated that no matter what type of play – constructive, outdoor, physical, or cooperative – play helps children learn and developmentally thrive, and the health and productivity of a child's play greatly affects later learning. Moor (2008) proposed that play with neurodivergent children can include relationship and structure. In the play context, choice, freedom, and discovery are simply not the only things that may motivate neurodivergent children to play in the way that they motivate neurotypical peers. Neurodivergent children may need structure as part of their play process. There may be anxiety, dysregulation, and needs for routine that would require a more structured/guided approach led by an affirming practitioner.

Play therapy and play interventions can be appropriate in working with Autistic and other neurodivergent children who have a variety of mental health needs (Parker and O'Brien, 2011). Play therapy approaches are gaining more and more valid research as effective therapy approaches for neurodivergent children and adolescents. Play interventions of many types – outdoor, movement, art, music, games, and prop based – provide the opportunity for the practitioner to individualize therapy and engage the child in both playful and structured approaches that validate the child's play preferences and interests.

Therapeutic Powers of Play

Schaefer and Drewes (2014) presented the therapeutic powers of play to deepen the knowledge of the core healing powers of play. Play is not just a

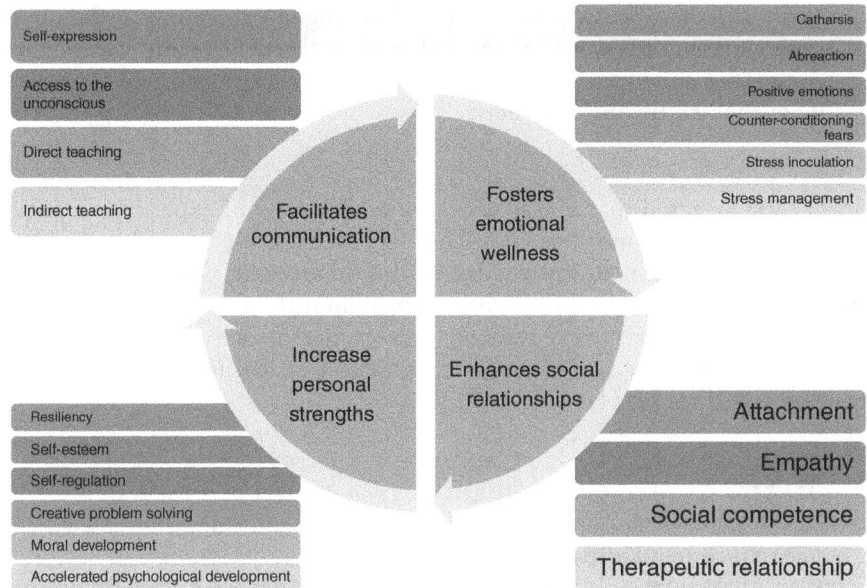

Figure 5.1 The therapeutic powers of play.
Stone, J. (2020). Adapted from Schaefer, C. E., & Drewes, A. A. (2013)

medium or context for applying other interventions, but that inherent in play behaviors is a broad spectrum of active forces that produce behavior change. When working with neurodivergent children, practitioners may focus in isolation or in combination on the specific powers of play. The twenty core agents of change of the therapeutic powers of play include: self-expression, access to the unconscious, direct teaching, indirect teaching, catharsis, abreaction, positive emotions, counterconditioning fears, stress inoculation, stress management, therapeutic relationship, attachment, social competence, empathy, creative problem-solving, resiliency, moral development, accelerated psychological development, self-regulation, and self-esteem. Figure 5.1 presents a visualization of the therapeutic powers of play.

Stone (2022) noted that the practitioner can utilize the structure of the therapeutic powers of play as a way to define what is being experienced within a session. Stone furthered that:

> The therapeutic powers are organized into four major categories: facilitate communication, foster emotional wellness, enhance social relationships, and increase personal strengths. These four categories are then described in more detail through the core agents of change as they are assigned to each category. A play therapist could recognize that a dynamic within the play intervention (client-tool, client-therapist, client-therapist-tool) enhanced social relationships, for example. To describe this dynamic further the therapist could choose from the core agents

under the therapeutic power of play heading. As an example, the discussion and/or notes would then explain that the play therapy session met the goal of enhanced social relationships, and the appropriate core agents were enacted through the play.

(p. 53)

Grant (2023) stated that it is likely the practitioner will experience a variety of the therapeutic powers of play. Thus, it becomes important for the therapist to have a grounded knowledge in the therapeutic powers of play. The intersection between the therapeutic powers and the therapist's understanding of the neurodiversity paradigm creates the most beneficial, safe, and healthy environment for neurodivergent children to address their mental health needs through play therapy.

References

Association for Play Therapy (2023). Definition of play therapy. https://www.a4pt.org/general/custom.asp?page=AboutAPT

Crenshaw, D., Stewart, A. L. & Brown, S. (2015). *Play therapy: A comprehensive guide to theory and practice*. Guilford.

Cross, A. (2010). *Come and play: Sensory integration strategies for children with play challenges*. Redleaf Press.

Grant, R. J. (2023). *The AutPlay therapy handbook: Integrative family play therapy with neurodivergent children*. Routledge.

Landreth, G. L. (1991). *Play therapy: The art of the relationship*. Psychology Press.

Moor, J. (2008). *Playing, laughing and learning with children on the autism spectrum*. Jessica Kingsley Publishers.

Parker, N. & O'Brien, P. (2011). Play therapy reaching the child with autism, *International Journal of Special Education*, 26, 80–87.

Phillips, N. & Beavan, L. (2010). *Teaching play to children with autism*. Thousand Oaks: Sage Publications.

Schaefer, C. E. & Drewes, A. A. (2014). *The therapeutic power of play: 20 core agents of change*. Wiley.

Sherratt, D. & Peter, M. (2002). *Developing play and drama in children with autistic spectrum disorders*. Fulton.

Stone, J. (2022). *Digital play therapy: A clinician's guide to comfort and competence*. Routledge.

Thornton, K. & Cox, E. (2005). Play and the reduction of challenging behavior in children with ASDs and learning disabilities. *Good Autism Practice*. 6:2, 75–80.

6 The Role of the Practitioner and the Parent

The Role of the Practitioner

The practitioner working with neurodivergent children and adolescents has multiple points of consideration. One of the primary roles is providing a neuro-diversity-affirming presence for the child. This process is covered more thoroughly in Chapter 1. The practitioner is always neurodiversity-affirming. Affirming should be evident in the intake process, in building the relationship with the child, in implementing play interventions, in the general ways the practitioner interacts with the child, and how the practitioner views the child. The practitioner will also need to make sure that any play approaches and interventions that are implemented with the child contain affirming and non-ableist concepts and messages. This process is covered more thoroughly in Chapter 4.

The practitioner is continually in the process of building the therapeutic relationship with the child and the parents. This concept is discussed in more detail in Chapter 2. Relationship development begins as soon as the practitioner makes any contact with the child and parents and is attended to throughout therapy until termination. It should be considered a foundation piece of therapy and understood to be one of the therapeutic powers of play. As play interventions are implemented, the practitioner should be aware that relationship development principles can still be implemented while participating in structured interventions.

The practitioner will set the stage for understanding the neurodivergent presentation of the child which will inform the play approaches and interventions that the practitioner will implement. For example, understanding the child's play preferences will help the practitioner select play interventions that match the child's preferences. Understanding the child's social navigation and communication style will help determine a more nondirective vs a directive approach, and in the selection of play therapy theory to help address the therapy goals.

Neurodivergent children and adolescents will present on a wide continuum regarding strengths, support needs, and awareness to complete various structured play interventions. The practitioner should be aware of this variance and be prepared to meet each child and adolescent where they are in terms of support needs. The practitioner's involvement in the facilitation,

DOI: 10.4324/9781003398691-6

completion, and processing of any intervention will depend on the needs of the child. Practitioners should be prepared for their involvement to be anywhere from very directive and involved in providing instruction and stopping to explain instructions or processes, to primarily being an observer and letting the child complete and process an intervention completely on their own.

Practitioners should always assume competence and let the child complete and process through any intervention as much as the child is capable. Thus, if the practitioner is unaware of the child's capability, then they should first let the child try before assuming the child is not capable and the practitioner needs to be involved in assisting the child. If a child is having difficulties completing an intervention, the practitioner should become more involved and guide the child through the intervention, breaking it down step by step if necessary.

Practitioners should be prepared to adapt their style and level of involvement at any time during a session and a play intervention. A neurodivergent child may be able to complete an intervention entirely on their own, not be able to complete any of the intervention without assistance from the practitioner, or complete part of an intervention but then become stuck at some point and need assistance from the practitioner. A willingness and flexibility to adjust from observer to participator to teacher is a key quality for the practitioner implementing structured play interventions with children. In summary, the practitioner must be comfortable being what the child needs.

The Role of the Parent

The Centers for Disease Control and Prevention (2023) stated that psychological therapy is meant to address a mental health condition or help a child manage their symptoms so that they can function well at home, in school, and in their community. When children are young, it is common for therapy to include the parent. Sometimes therapists work with the parents alone. Older children may meet with a therapist alone as well. Some types of therapy include working with the whole family or other important adults in the child's life (for example, a teacher). Parent-focused approaches typically mean that parents talk with the therapist about the child's behavior and feelings. Therapists may also observe parents and children together and then make suggestions for finding different ways to react.

Booth and Jernberg (2010) stated that a secure attachment relationship is both the outcome of healthy parent—child interaction and the key to long-term mental health. Such a relationship is just as important in helping the neurodivergent child achieve optimal mental health goals as it is with the neurotypical child. Further, when parents are part of the therapy, they carry on the successful interactions with the child at home. Home interactions provide the added benefit that the child can generalize from the therapy setting to the home.

Therapy approaches involving neurodivergent children typically include parent participation and/or a training component. The level of parent involvement can vary, and potential options include regular consultations between the practitioner and the parents, formal parent training, family play sessions where the parent and child participate together, and parents being taught to implement therapy approaches at home with their child. Grant (2017) proposed that parents are the people most knowledgeable about their children and the most equipped with the opportunities to assist their children in everyday situations. Parent involvement empowers parents to become co-change agents and a sustainable resource for supporting the neurodivergent child's mental health needs.

Seminal play therapy approaches include parent involvement at a variety of levels from consultations to full family play therapy (Landreth, 1991; VanFleet, 2014; Jernberg and Booth, 2001). AutPlay Therapy protocol is adjustable to involve parents are various levels (Grant, 2023). The practitioner and parents may schedule periodic consultation meetings to provide updates, the practitioner may meet with the parents at the beginning of each session for a parent update, the practitioner may establish that several sessions of parent-focused training would be helpful, or the practitioner may fully involve the parents participating with the child in sessions and implementing play interventions at home. The play interventions in this book are designed to be taught to parents and for parents to implement the interventions at home between therapy sessions.

Practitioners planning to implement a parent training component should establish clear guidelines for what is to be covered and how it relates to the identified therapy goals. Practitioners who are implementing full family play therapy involvement, which includes in-home processes, will want to monitor home implementation carefully to make sure play interventions are being implemented at home accurately and successfully. Further, parents will likely have several questions throughout the process of therapy, and sufficient time should be allowed to thoroughly address any parent questions or concern.

References

Booth, P. B., & Jernberg, A. M. (2010). *Theraplay: Helping parents and children build better relationships through attachment-based play*. Jossey Bass.

Centers for Disease Control and Prevention (2023). Therapy to improve children's mental health. https://www.cdc.gov/childrensmentalhealth/parent-behavior-therapy.html

Grant, R. J. (2017). *AutPlay therapy for children and adolescents on the autism spectrum: A behavioral play-based approach*. Routledge.

Grant, R. J. (2023). *The AutPlay therapy handbook: Integrative family play therapy with neurodivergent children*. Routledge.

Jernberg, A. M., & Booth, P. B. (2001). *Theraplay: Helping parents and children build better relationships through attachment-based play*. New Jersey: John Wiley and Sons Inc.

Landreth, G. L. (1991). *Play therapy: The art of the relationship*. Accelerated Development Inc. Publishers.

VanFleet, R. (2014). *Filial therapy: Strengthening parent-child relationships through play*. Professional Resource Press.

7 Social Navigation Interventions

Collaborative Painting

Therapy Needs: Connection, engagement, relationship development, social navigation needs (completing a task together)	
Level: Child, adolescent	
Materials: Paper, paint (can also be done with paper and markers)	
Modality: Individual, family, and group	

Introduction

Applicable for working with neurodivergent children and adolescents who have therapy needs related to connection and engagement with others, working with others to complete a task, and participating in (and accomplishing) an activity together in a positive relationship-building manner. This intervention is most appropriate for children who have a play preference or special interest in art and/or expressive experiences.

Instructions

1) The practitioner explains to the child/adolescent that they are going to create a painting together.
2) The practitioner tells the child that the child will go first and start painting something (the child does not tell the practitioner what they are painting, and the practitioner and child do not decide on a picture ahead of time).
3) The child can have an idea in mind or just randomly begin painting but they do not share what they are thinking with the practitioner.
4) The practitioner times the child for one minute then says, 'Switch'. The practitioner then has one minute to add to the picture while the child

DOI: 10.4324/9781003398691-7

times the practitioner for one minute. The practitioner is adding to the picture but also not telling the child what they are thinking.

5) When the minute is up, the child says, 'Switch'. This goes back and forth until it seems like the picture is at an end point.

6) When it seems the picture is at an end point, the practitioner can check with the child and if both agree, they can end. The amount of time it takes to complete a painting varies, but there is usually an obvious stopping point. The child and practitioner then discuss what they made together, and each put their signature on the painting.

Rationale

This play intervention helps children and adolescents work on connection and relationship development, as well as social navigation related to taking turns, cooperating, and working together to complete a task. It is offered in a playful way that ideally taps into the child's play preferences. The practitioner might discuss with the child how it feels to work with someone else to make something, especially when you do not get to choose how everything goes. Parents can be taught how to do this intervention at home and encouraged to create several collaborative paintings with their child. Parents and child can also bring their collaborative paintings to sessions and show the practitioner.

Merry Go Build aka Pass the Base

(Contributed by Tony Vallance, Child Play Therapist)

Therapy Needs: Social navigation needs, perspective taking, understanding of empathic responses.
Level: Child, adolescent
Materials: Enough LEGO® base plates for participants, LEGO® bricks (in open, accessible tubs), a table to work at.
Modality: Group, family

Introduction

Autistic and other neurodivergent individuals, as well as neurotypical children, may require support to develop their capacity to understand and navigate their thoughts, emotions, and desires and those of others around them (especially when they may be different). This play therapy intervention is designed to build a child's ability to understand and regulate around the process of working together to create and appreciate others' ideas. This can be a useful integrative group idea as many neurotypical children could also benefit from accepting the process and ideas of neurodivergent children.

Instructions

1) Participants will sit around a table or in a circle on the floor.
2) They are each given a blank LEGO® base plate and instructed the following. 'For this activity we are learning how to share ideas and build on them... literally using LEGO®. You each will be given a LEGO® base plate and, using the LEGO® bricks in the tubs, create any design, shape, or object you want. You only have three minutes though and after that time is up, you are to pass the base plate to the person sitting on the right next to you. Then, with the new LEGO® creation in front of you, you are to keep building on top of what you now have.'
3) The children begin and after three minutes the therapist reminds them it is time to pass their bass plate to the person on their right and continue to build.
4) After three minutes is up again, the therapist instructs the children to pass their bass plate to the person on their right once more. This will keep happening every three minutes until the original base plate is in front of the original child.
5) For this activity, the children can only build on designs, not remove blocks, as the focus is own creativity accepting, building on ideas, and accomplishing together.
6) Once the activity has been completed, the children can share about what their bass plate now looks like and how they might think or feel about the process and changes.
7) Music can be nice to add in the background if sensorially appropriate for all the participants.

Rationale

This play intervention utilizes a common play preference of neurodivergent children – LEGO® bricks. It targets the development of perspective and acceptance for participants in that they will be building on the creative expressions of others. They will engage with the LEGO® bricks in a tactile and creative way, which will help to reinforce the concept that everybody has their own way of doing things.

Friend Collage

Therapy Needs: Social navigation, friendship-related needs
Level: Child, adolescent
Materials: Paper, several magazines, markers, pen or pencil
Modality: Individual, group

Introduction

Friendship navigation can be a common concern, issue, or questioning place for many neurodivergent children and adolescents. This play intervention helps children explore what activities they would like to do and feel comfortable doing with other children. This intervention encourages application by having the practitioner play out scenarios with the child to help them feel confident and reduce any possible anxiety related to peer interactions. The practitioner will need several magazines for the child to look through. Magazines that have a child focus will likely be more beneficial. Affirming note: friendships for neurodivergent children can have a look and feel that works for them. It does not have to be the way you think it should look or feel. Friendship goals should be a need the child expresses and wants help with. If the child is fine with how their friendship world is operating, then that should be respected.

Instructions

1) The child draws a person figure (outline) on a piece of paper. The outline should be large and cover most of the paper.
2) The child is then instructed to cut out from magazines several pictures and/or words of things they like to do and play preferences/interests they have, especially ones they think they might like to do with another person. If the child is struggling to identify things they can do with other children, the practitioner can help the child think of ideas.
3) The child glues all the cut-outs on and around the person figure drawn on the piece of paper.
4) The child creates a collage of all the activities that they have identified that could be done with another person. Figure 7.1 presents an example of a completed Friend Collage.
5) The practitioner and child go through each of the activities and talk about them together.
6) The child is welcome to identify a real child who might be appropriate to do each activity with and discuss how they can begin to initiate completing the activity with the child.
7) If appropriate, the practitioner and child decide on an activity that the child will try to do with another person before their next session, and the practitioner and child can play out the activity together for practice. The play-out practice can be helpful for increasing confidence and decreasing anxiety.

Rationale

This play intervention helps children and adolescents work on social navigation, specifically related to friendship desires and needs. This intervention can also help address possible anxiety issues related to peer contact. Affirming

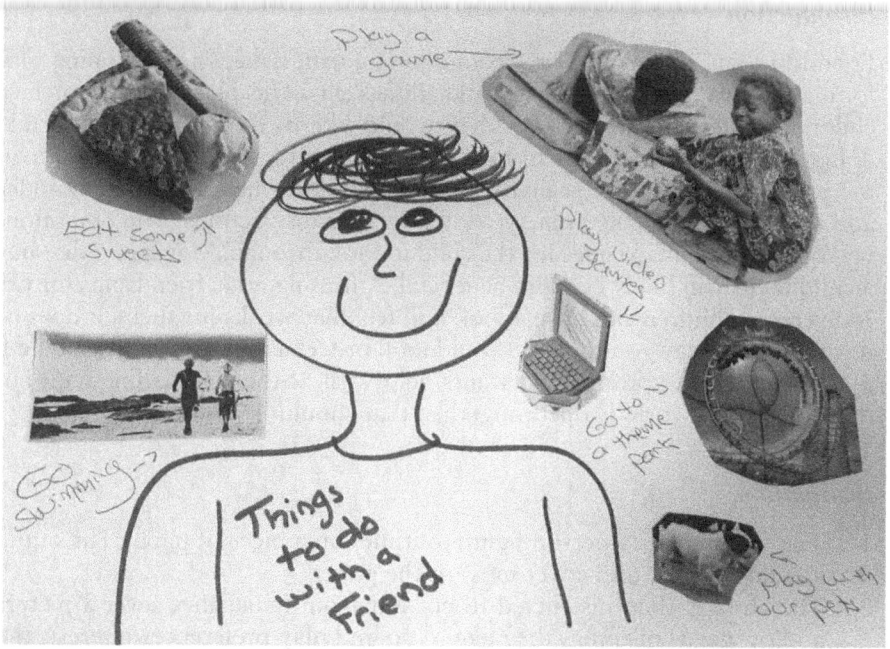

Figure 7.1 Completed 'Friend Collage'.

Robert Jason Grant

note: some children are not safe and some neurotypical children may not understand or appreciate the neurodivergent child. This may need to be discussed as part of this activity, especially if the child wants to try and initiate with a particular child. The parents may also need to be a part of this activity for understanding and implementation.

Social Safety Scales

Therapy Needs: Social navigation, safety-related issues
Level: Child, adolescent
Materials: Paper, pencil, various created social situations
Modality: Individual, group

Introduction

Social safety scales intervention is designed to help practitioners create specific scenarios in which a child or adolescent might need help in developing or understanding better or more appropriate social responses in safety scenarios. The sample scales provided can be used as a guide, but scales should be created to address the safety needs of the child the practitioner is seeing. The scales can be used as both an assessment tool to identify what the child understands and an intervention tool to help develop social safety awareness.

Instructions

1) The practitioner creates a scales sheet with several scales listed on it. The practitioner can create several scenarios to use the scales as an assessment tool to discover what the child understands about safety. The therapist can also create a set of scales specific to things the child is struggling with that they need to better understand. Practitioners should write scales considering the age and cognitive level of the child. Practitioners can read the scales to children who cannot read and they can also use visuals.
2) The child is given the scales sheet and the first situation is read. The child puts an X on the scale where they believe is the correct response for the situation.
3) Once the child has given a response, the child's response should be processed with the practitioner. The practitioner should especially discuss any response that seems unhealthy, unsafe, or not accurate. An example might be the practitioner reads, 'A stranger walks up to you while you are at the mall or playing at a park and says if you come with me, I can get you a free iPad. Mark on the scale where you think this would fall on the truth and lie scale and the safe and unsafe scale.' Wherever the child marks can be discussed but especially if the child were to mark near the truth or safe end of the scale. This might require some repeated psychoeducation.

Example scale

Truth--Lie

Safe--Not Safe

4) This intervention can be repeated in various sessions. It is usually helpful for children to periodically review social safety issues to make sure they retain information in their memory and processing.

Rationale

It is well documented that Autistic and other neurodivergent children are highly susceptible to abuse and victimization. This play intervention incorporates more psychoeducation processes to help teach children and adolescents safety awareness. Practitioners are encouraged to utilize their own creativity and adjust the intervention to make it as playful as possible. Parents can be involved in this intervention and encouraged to support safety awareness education at home.

Example Situations and Scales

You are sitting in class at school and the boy beside you starts hitting his desk.
Safe---Not Safe

You are walking down the hallway at school and another student pushes you as you pass by.
Bullying---Not Bullying

You meet a new student at school and talk for a few minutes about her old school.
Safe---Not Safe

A student at school says your hair looks like an anime character.
Bullying---Not Bullying

Another student at school who has been nice to you asks you to show them your private parts.
Okay---Not Okay

A student at school says he will be your friend if you keep his vape for him.
Safe---Not Safe
Friend--Not a Friend

Celebrating Questions

Therapy Needs: Social navigation, asking questions
Level: Child and adolescent
Materials: Some type of celebratory item – candy, stickers, pebbles, pencils, balloons, pennies, small toys (rings, balls, animals), etc.
Modality: Individual, group

Introduction

Neurodivergent children can often experience anxiety when needing to ask questions, especially in a public setting and with those who they are not familiar with. This play intervention helps children and adolescents work on asking other people questions. The celebrating item serves as a fun and playful element to help relax children and keep them engaged.

Instructions

1) The practitioner will have available one or more celebratory items that the child can choose as they complete the intervention.

2) The practitioner should try to choose items that the child likes and also consider if the child has any special diet restrictions (if including candy or another type of food).

3) The practitioner tells the child they are going to play celebrating questions to help the child feel more comfortable asking questions.

4) The practitioner is going to start by providing the child with a list of questions to ask the practitioner. This should begin with simple questions like 'Do you like pets?' or 'What is your favorite video game?' As the child can ask the practitioner a question, the child picks a celebratory item to keep. One celebratory item for each question asked.

5) As the child can ask questions, the practitioner can provide another list with typical scenarios from the child's life where they may need to ask a question such as 'Where is the bathroom?' or 'I did not hear you, can you repeat that?' The child then has to ask the practitioner these questions, the practitioner will answer, and the child can choose a celebratory item.

6) The practitioner can have many questions ready to share and can also turn the process over to the child and they can ask any question they want – something they are wondering about, or something from their daily life.

7) This intervention does not have to be done verbally: questions can be written, a device can be used to ask questions, and visuals or any other method can be incorporated. This will depend on the child and their communication style.

Rationale

Neurodivergent children can struggle with anxiety, fear, and other barriers that prevent them from being able to ask important questions. This play intervention is designed to help children and adolescents become more confident and less anxious about asking questions. It would be beneficial for the practitioner to have a pre-determined set of questions written out to ask the child before the child's session. The practitioner can play the intervention with the child several times and in various sessions to help reduce anxiety and to support question asking in the child's daily life. Parents can be included in this intervention and can play at home with their child. Parents may experience more opportunities to play the intervention in real-life scenarios and help the child gain confidence.

Friend Mapping

Therapy Needs: Social navigation, friendship issues
Level: Child, adolescent
Materials: Friend Mapping Worksheet (available in the Appendix), pen or pencil
Modality: Individual

Introduction

Children and adolescents can struggle with understanding friendships and differentiating friends from acquaintances from 'frenemies'. This intervention helps children better identify what healthy friendship looks like for them and also serves as an assessment tool in helping the practitioner gain a better understanding of what is happening in regard to the child's peer/friend relationships.

Instructions

1) The practitioner tells the child that they are going to work on discussing and identifying friendships.
2) Using the Friend Mapping Worksheet (located in the Appendix), the child is instructed to complete each section. In the circles, the child will write the names of three current friends, three things they do with friends, three things the child does with other children of the same age, and three people that they would like to be friends with.
3) In the two rectangles, the child will write two things that make a good friendship.
4) The practitioner will then process through the map with the child asking follow-up questions to gain a better understating of the child's current reality and perceptions of friendships.
5) If the child is struggling to identify any areas of the friendship map, the practitioner should provide assistance to the child.
6) The practitioner should provide affirming information throughout the process. The child can navigate friendship in the way that feels most comfortable for them. They do not have to 'fit' some preconceived society standard.
7) This intervention is primarily designed to help children better understand and meet their friendship goals and to better understand a friend from someone who is not being a friend.

Rationale

Friend mapping is an intervention that helps children and adolescents work on social navigation, specifically related to peer relationships and friendships. Children can need help in differentiating between relationship levels (friend vs not treating me well) and help in creating and participating in friendships. This intervention also serves as an assessment tool for practitioners to gain a clearer understanding of the child's current friendship world and the child's perception of what constitutes a friend. Practitioners will likely begin and end this intervention with a discussion of what friendship can look like and what feels most comfortable for the child – the various options which include in-person and online friends and various levels of satisfaction in friendship interactions.

Paper Friend

Therapy Needs: Social navigation, friendship issues	
Level: Child, adolescent	
Materials: White paper, construction paper, scissors, glue	
Modality: Individual	

Introduction

This play intervention provides an expressive and visual construction designed to help children address friendship-related wants and needs, specifically targeting children to engage with on a friendship level, and strategies to help develop and maintain friendships. Affirming note: many neurodivergent children will have a preferred way they interact with and define meaningful friendships. This should be understood and respected. The practitioner will work with the child to help them achieve any friendship-related goals that are important to the child.

Instructions

1) The practitioner explains to the child that they will be talking about friendships.
2) The practitioner or child draws an outline of a person on a white piece of paper.
3) The child identifies someone in their life that they would like to be friends with or get to know better.
4) The child designs the person outline to look like the child they would like to be friends with (typically by drawing the identified child's face on the paper outline person).
5) The child then writes things on the person outline that they could do with that person, things they could talk about, ways they could interact, ways that they could initiate with that person, and what they think would make that person a good friend. The practitioner can write for the child and can discuss these concepts with the child and share suggestions.
6) The practitioner and child process through what the child has written.
7) The practitioner and child can practice (role-play) some of the identified ideas.
8) This may be an ongoing intervention that is revisited through several sessions, especially if the child has a great deal of anxiety about interacting with peers. Further, if the child identifies a real person they would like to engage with, the practitioner should verify though parents (or other sources) that this would be an appropriate child. Some peers may not be safe (or appropriate for another reason) and we do not want the child attempting something that could harm them.

Rationale

Peer navigation and friendship can be stressful, confusing, and troubling for many neurodivergent children. This play intervention can help children and adolescents address friendship-related wants and needs. It provides the opportunity to better understand the child and their preferences when it comes to friendships. It also provides the opportunity to help the child connect with other children who may have similar interests and play styles.

Bully in the Way

Therapy Needs: Social navigation, addressing bullying issues
Level: Child, adolescent
Materials: White paper, markers, small prize
Modality: Individual

Introduction

It is well documented that Autistic and other neurodivergent children are highly susceptible to being bullied. This play intervention is designed to help children and adolescents understand bullying situations and to role-play/practice what to do and say if someone is trying to bully them.

Instructions

1) The practitioner explains to the child that they are going to discuss ways to address bullying behavior.
2) The practitioner and child draw and cut out several people shapes. The child decorates each person shape to represent a real person who has bullied the child (if the child cannot think of real people, then fictious bullies can be used).
3) Once the child is finished, each of the 'bullies' are placed on the floor scattered from one side of the room to the other side.
4) The practitioner discusses with the child how each person that the child has made has bullied them or, with fictious people, how they might bully others.
5) The child then starts at one side of the room, walks up to each bully, confronts that bully, and practices a helpful response or action that they could give to that bully. The practitioner may have to teach the child various responses or actions that the child could take. Table 7.1 provides some examples for addressing bullying.
6) The child confronts each bully one at a time until they get through all the bullies and the child is on the other side of the room.

Table 7.1 Bully in the Way

Example interventions to implement:
Tell the school counselor or teacher
Tell your parents
Teach positive cognition statements to say to self
Leave the situation
Teach self-worth concepts to improve self-esteem
Keep a journal of the bullying
Work with the school to create a peer assignment program
Stay with friends
Ignore the bully
Teach comeback phrases (if child is capable)
Talk loudly back to the bully (if child is capable)
Call the bully by their name and tell them to stop (if child is capable)

Source: Grant, R. J. (2023).

7) After the last bully has been confronted, the child receives a small prize provided by the practitioner (prizes are optional but can be fun and celebratory for the child).

Rationale

Statistics highlight that neurodivergent children are more susceptible to bullying and victimization than their neurotypical peers. Often neurodivergent children are unsure how to navigate a bullying situation. If bullying experiences are left unaddressed, it can result in significant mental health issues. This play technique helps children and adolescents begin to understand how to address bullying. Affirming note: Bullying is not simply the child's responsibility to address. The practitioner will likely need to discuss bullying problems with parents, who will likely need to contact the school if bullying is happening at school and make the school administration aware of the bullying. Both parents and school officials may need to be involved in eliminating the bullying. Bullying situations should not be dismissed by adults as typical kid behavior, and the practitioner may have to advocate for the child and hold the adults in charge accountable to following through with a solution.

Social Media

Therapy Needs: Social navigation, understanding social media experiences	
Level: Child, adolescent	
Materials: Computer, tablet or smartphone, social media account	
Modality: Individual, group	

Introduction

Social media sites are very popular among children and adolescents. This play intervention is designed to teach children and adolescents how to identify appropriate/safe and inappropriate/unsafe ways to navigate through and use social media sites and how to stay safe with their interactions with other people.

Instructions

1) The practitioner tells the child that they will be discussing navigating and using various social media sites. The practitioner should inquire if the child currently has any social media sites they use. Before implementing this intervention, the practitioner should also discuss with parents if the child currently has any social media accounts and/or if they are planning to allow the child to have one.

2) The practitioner and child discuss the various social media options including whatever sites the child may navigate and sites other children often use (Facebook, Twitter, Snapchat, Discord, Instagram, YouTube, etc.)

3) The following acronym is written down on a piece of paper:
   F=friend
   A=angry
   C=careful
   E=embarrassing
   B=bad
   O=odd
   O=oh no!
   K=kind

4) The practitioner and child discuss what different Facebook posts (any social media account could be used) would look like for each of the above categories. For example: Who is a friend? Why is that person a friend? What is an angry post? Is it appropriate to post angry things? What would be an embarrassing post? What would be odd or bad to post? What is a post that could get someone in trouble or is unsafe? And what is a kind or appropriate post? The practitioner and child try to find examples of each one on the child and/or practitioner's Facebook (or other social media) newsfeed.

5) Ideally the practitioner and child would be viewing an account the child has. The practitioner can also print off selected posts from their own account (prior to the child's session) to use as examples to discuss.

Rationale

Children and adolescents engage in various social media accounts and interactions daily. This can provide a wonderful way to interact with others, make friends, and gain information. It can also be very problematic for a variety of reasons. This play intervention helps children be prepared for participating in and socializing through social media. This play intervention requires the child to have a social media account or be in the process of creating one. The practitioner should also discuss with parents about monitoring their child's social media accounts and periodically reviewing/practicing this intervention at home with their child.

Tweet Tweet Tweet

Therapy Needs: Social navigation, social media education
Level: Adolescent
Materials: Paper, pencil, example tweets
Modality: Individual, group

Introduction

Adolescents are typically exposed to social media and often have a difficult time navigating appropriateness and safety through media formats. This play intervention helps adolescents practice what appropriate/safe and inappropriate/unsafe social media responses look like on Twitter. This intervention can be done using any social media platform.

Instructions

1) The practitioner explains to the adolescent that they will be discussing appropriate and inappropriate social media comments.
2) The practitioner and child then role-play sending appropriate and inappropriate/unsafe messages back and forth to each other.
3) The child should be able to identify the appropriate from the inappropriate/unsafe and why the inappropriate messages are considered inappropriate.
4) The practitioner then gives the adolescent several real tweets taken from Twitter (Table 7.2 provides several examples) and the adolescent must put them in two piles: one pile is for appropriate tweets, and the other pile is for inappropriate or unsafe tweets. The child must talk about why

Table 7.2 Example Tweets

Develop an attitude of #gratitude and give thanks for everything that happens to you.
Lol no one likes you.
MERRY CHRISTMAS to the members and families of the Ozark Drumline!
Friday afternoon will be warm and sunny, colder weekend.
So are you straight or gay I'm like really confused.
F#%k my mom she deletes my fb dat b#%*h can go die.
I hate you, Ted.
You and me. Lunch next week. I won't be late this time.
That's like saying Superman is better than Batman. You're dead to me.
Just finished doing laundry. I hate Laundry!
Congratulations! Your new baby is so cute!!!!!
This is a great website for information on bully prevention.
She is a complete slut! I hate her!!! HATE!!!
I am seriously going to kill someone if all these a#%es don't stop messing with me.
The Hobbit is an awesome movie! Just saw it – Loved It!
Really frustrated with everything right now.
Guess who is on TV acting like a total retard!?!
Home alone, so bored. Somebody hit me up!

Source: Grant, R. J. (2023).

they think each tweet is either appropriate or inappropriate/unsafe. If the adolescent is unsure if the tweet is appropriate or inappropriate/unsafe, then they can make a third pile of unsure tweets and the practitioner and adolescent can further discuss those tweets. The practitioner should provide feedback and assist the child if they are labeling something as appropriate that could be unsafe.

5) The practitioner could also add to this intervention a discussion about what to do if someone sends or communicates to them something that is not appropriate or is unsafe.

Rationale

Social media exposure and usage are very common among adolescents. Often the usage comes with very little education about how the platforms and interactions can be unsafe. This play intervention helps adolescents work on identifying what would be inappropriate or unsafe to produce on social media. This intervention does not require the adolescent to have a Twitter or any other social media account. It is a good intervention to practice before a child acquires any social media account. The practitioner should discuss with parents the relevance of social media access in the adolescent's life before implementing this intervention. If the adolescent is currently using any social media site or is planning to, this would be an appropriate intervention to implement. This intervention can be taught to parents at home and parents can continue to implement this intervention periodically with their adolescent.

Role-play

Therapy Needs: Social navigation, social anxiety
Level: Child, adolescent
Materials: None
Modality: Individual, family, group

Introduction

Neurodivergent children may have anxiety related to various social situations they must navigate. Sometimes, the anxiety can be so intense that it will prevent the child from doing something they want or need to do. Practitioners can identify several situations where a child or adolescent may need help in reducing their social anxiety. The role-playing intervention provides opportunity to practice situations to reduce anxiety. The role-plays should be fun and engaging and can include props and other people.

Instructions

1) The practitioner explains to the child that they are going to role-play some situations the child has been having anxiety about. The practitioner should be aware of situations that produce anxiety for the child (parent and/or child reports) and target these situations specifically through the role-playing. This could be things like getting their hair cut, riding in a car, brushing their teeth, etc.
2) The practitioner and child will decide on what situations to role-play, who will be in each role, and if any props will be used. The role-plays should be fun and exaggerated.
3) Once the role-play is finished, it should be completed again with the practitioner and child switching roles. For example, if the practitioner was a hairdresser and the child was themselves in the first practice, then they would switch roles in the second practice.
4) Role-plays should be practiced several times throughout a session. Repetition and practice can be helpful for reducing anxiety. The more the child can role-play the anxiety-producing situations, the more likely they will be able to accomplish the task.
5) An added element would be to record one of the role-plays and have the child take the recording with them and watch it right before or as they are completing the real task.

6) Anxiety responses may be due to a sensory or trauma trigger or from a situation the child is entering being one that is unsafe (such as going to school and being consistently bullied). The practitioner should be aware of these other possible sources for the anxiety, which would require additional intervention efforts.

Rationale

High anxiety, especially regarding social navigation can be a common issue for neurodivergent children. This play intervention helps reduce anxiety through a role-play. When doing a role-play, it is best to avoid working in a metaphor or an approximate to the child's situation. Instead focus should be on directly talking about a specific situation that the child struggles with. Role-plays can be taught to parents and parents can practice the role-plays at home with their child. Parents can also role-play any situation that comes up that they feel needs attention.

Social Media: Friend, Foe, or Other

Therapy Needs: Social navigation, social media education
Level: Adolescent
Materials: Social media account, index cards, pencil
Modality: Individual, family, group

Introduction

Adolescents are often attracted to engaging with other people though social media as it provides a safe boundary and usually presents less social anxiety and better opportunities to connect with friends. This play intervention helps adolescents understand different levels of 'knowing' someone and safety-related awareness with meeting someone through a social media site.

Instructions

1) The practitioner explains to the adolescent that they are going to discuss being safe when interacting with others through social media. This intervention is best done with adolescents who have a social media account or are planning to start one.

2) The practitioner should discuss this intervention with parents before implementing it with the adolescent. The practitioner and adolescent go through the adolescent's friends or followers list on one of the adolescent's social media accounts. The adolescent identifies each person as a friend, a family member, an acquaintance, a stranger, or an enemy, and

tells the practitioner if they know the person in real life or through social media.

3) As the adolescent identifies, the practitioner writes the name down on an index card, how the adolescent labels the person, and if the adolescent knows the person in real life or through social media.

4) After each person has been covered, all the index cards are placed in categories according to how the adolescent identified the person. The practitioner and adolescent then go through each category and talk about the number of 'friends' in that category and the number of people the adolescent knows only through social media.

5) The practitioner and adolescent then discuss different levels of knowing people and possible safety concerns of interacting through social media with people that are only known online. Discussion items would include – Is this person really who they say they are? How would you know for certain? How do predators operate on social media? What types of information would you share and not share with this person?

Rationale

This play intervention is designed to help adolescents understand developing and navigating relationships acquired through social media in an educated and safe manner. This intervention also works on understanding different levels of knowing people and what constitutes a friend, someone you know well, an acquaintance, etc. It can also be discussed with parents how to monitor social media accounts and how to periodically use this intervention at home with their child.

Social Navigation Fortune Tellers

Therapy Needs: Social navigation needs and questions, anxiety reduction
Level: Child, adolescent
Materials: Paper, markers
Modality: Individual, family, group

Introduction

This play intervention provides a fun and engaging game for children to share social navigation questions and practice anxiety-producing social situations. The social-related questions and situations should be real things the child would like to process. The tactile and movement piece of the fortune teller provides an engaging and regulating component for the child, and many children find this intervention fun to create and do and want to create multiple fortune tellers.

Instructions

1) The practitioner explains to the child that they are going to be making paper fortune tellers and using the fortune tellers to explore social-related question and navigation needs.
2) The practitioner teaches the child how to make a fortune teller out of white paper or colored construction paper (instructions for the creation of a fortune teller can be found online).
3) Fortune tellers should have numbers on the outside, colors on the inside, and a social-related question or anxiety-producing situation written on the tab on the other side of each color (Figure 7.2 provides an example).
4) After the fortune teller has been created, the practitioner and child can take turns playing the game. The basic process of the game is as follows. The practitioner holds the fortune teller in their fingers. The child chooses a number, and the practitioner moves the fortune teller back and forth for the number of times that the child chose. The practitioner opens up the fortune teller and the child chooses a color. The practitioner lifts the tab for that color which reveals a question or a situation to practice. The practitioner and child then talk about the question or practice the situation.
5) The practitioner should let the child create questions and situations that are relevant for them. The practitioner may have to help the child but should make sure the social questions and situations chosen apply to the child.

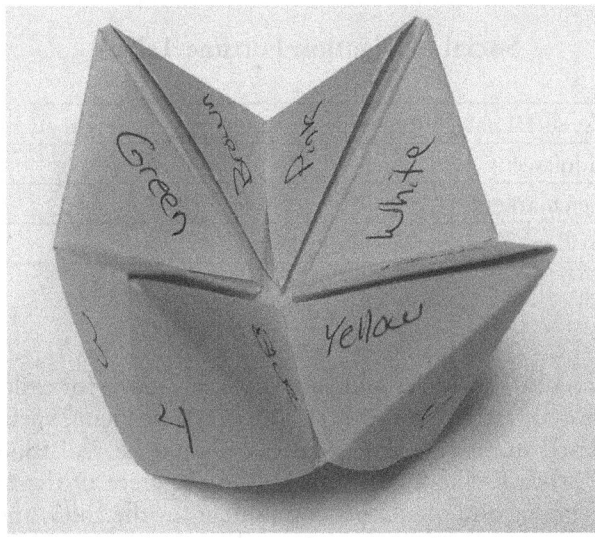

Figure 7.2 Fortune teller.

Robert Jason Grant

6) Once the fortune teller is complete, there should be eight social-related questions or situations written inside.

7) Affirming note: discussions and responses to questions and practicing social situations should stay affirming of the child. The practitioner is not trying to make the child look or act neurotypical. The practitioner is affirming of the child's identity and ways of interacting socially. The practitioner is implementing this activity to help the child conceptualize social navigation in a way that will work best for them to achieve what they desire.

Rationale

Neurodivergent children may have many questions about social navigation. They may also have certain social situations that create anxiety for them and in which they have a difficult time navigating. This play intervention helps children and adolescents address their questions and practice affirming navigation. More than one fortune teller can be made. The practitioner and child may create one that is just questions and one that is situations to practice. The child can take their fortune tellers home and play with other family members. Parents can be taught how to make fortune tellers at home and how to play the game with their children.

Three Foam Dice

Therapy Needs: Social navigation, relationship development
Level: Child, adolescent
Materials: Foam dice, markers
Modality: Individual, family, group

Introduction

Three foam dice is a play intervention that focuses on positive interactions with another person and deepening relationship development. Three large foam dice are used in a game format to allow for the practitioner and child to engage in a variety of ways.

Instructions

1) Using three foam dice, the practitioner designates one of the dice to be something to ask the other person, one to be something to share about self, and one to be an activity to do together.

2) The practitioner may have dice already made or they can be made with the child. Dice 1 has something to ask the other person, and something is written on each side of the dice such as, what colors do you like? What are your favorite video games? What have you eaten this week?

Dice 2 has something to share about yourself and something is written on each side, such as my favorite video game, what I like to do for fun, how many people are in my family, etc.

Dice 3 has an activity to do together and something is written on each side, such as hop around the room, thumb wrestle, blow some bubbles, etc.

3) The child rolls all three dice and whatever is displayed on the upside of each dice is what the child and therapist will do and the number on the dice is the number of times they will do it. For example: if the child rolls dice 1 and it is a 3 with the question, 'What have you eaten this week?', the practitioner and child will each have to say three things they have eaten that week. After all three dice are completed that the child rolled, the practitioner will then roll the dice.

4) The practitioner and child continue to roll the dice and play the intervention until they have implemented everything written on the dice or until the practitioner or child ends the game.

Rationale

Neurodivergent children may have a play preference for game play. This play intervention works on multiple social and engaging processes simultaneously. When creating the dice, practitioners should consider the individual child that they will be working with – their age, accommodations, and any disability needs they may have. Foam dice come in various sizes and can be found online and in most educational supply stores. The foam dice can be given to the child to take home and parents and other family members can play with the child.

School Days

Therapy Needs: Social navigation, school-related issues, anxiety
Level: Child, adolescent
Materials: Paper, markers, highlighters
Modality: Individual, group

Introduction

Arguably, the school setting is the largest social setting that the child participates in and is often the most anxiety-producing and dysregulating environment due to the myriad of social situations, sensory experiences, transitions, etc. School Days helps the child identify various social and other dynamics that the child may encounter and how to navigate social situations and other dynamics presented during a given school day. This intervention can also serve as an assessment tool to help identify what struggles are happening at school and possible accommodations the child may need.

Instructions

1) The practitioner explains to the child that they will be working on identifying school-related situations that may feel uncomfortable or anxiety-producing for the child.
2) The child draws a picture of their school on a piece of paper.
3) The child writes on or around the school any of the things related to school that make them feel anxious, scared, or confused.
4) The child then draws another picture of their school and on or around the school, they write anything that they like about school.
5) The practitioner and child go through each school drawing and talk about what the child created.
6) The practitioner will want to assess what sems problematic for the child and how to best help the child with these issues. The practitioner may design interventions to help the child and/or may need to advocate for accommodations or changes to the child's school day.

Rationale

School can produce many issues for a neurodivergent child and most schools are not set up to value or allow for a neurodivergent child's preferred and comfortable way of learning and navigating. This play intervention works on identifying the struggles a child is having with school days and what can be done to help the child. Parents may be involved in this intervention to help advocate for any accommodations or changes that may need to be made to the child's school experience.

8 Feeling Identification and Expression Interventions

My Feeling World

Therapy Needs: Feeling identification and expression, regulation, and connection
Level: Child, adolescent
Materials: Paper, markers, tape
Modality: Individual, group

Introduction

This intervention is designed to help children recognize feelings that they experience in specific situations. This intervention can be used as a regulation and assessment tool to identify a child's level of emotional regulation and identify specific environments that create negative feelings for the child.

Instructions

1) The practitioner and child decide upon four different environments that the child experiences, such as school, home, scouts, soccer practice, dance class, church, etc.
2) The practitioner and child write each of the four places on different pieces of paper and tape each piece of paper in different corners around the playroom.
3) The practitioner and child each get a different color of marker. The practitioner explains to the child that they are going to take a trip to each of the places; the child decides where they are going to go first.
4) The practitioner and child walk to that piece of paper and both the practitioner and child write on the piece of paper a positive feeling and a negative feeling about that place.
5) Both the practitioner and child then talk about why they have those feelings.

DOI: 10.4324/9781003398691-8

6) The practitioner and child then travel to the next place and complete the same process until all four places have been visited. Once all four have been completed, the child receives a small prize. The prize is optional but can be fun and celebratory for completing the intervention.

Rationale

Feeling identification and emotional regulation can be a challenge for any child. This play intervention helps children work on identifying feelings and increasing emotional regulation ability. The focus is on helping a child identify feelings they experience in different settings in their life and being able to express why they experience the feelings. The intervention can be repeated with new environments.

Musical Feelings

Therapy Needs: Feeling identification and expression, regulation, and connection
Level: Child, adolescent
Materials: Several music instruments
Modality: Individual, group

Introduction

This play intervention teaches feeling identification and emotional regulation by introducing a musical element that can be engaging and provide an additional sensory-satisfying element. Before introducing this intervention, the practitioner would want to know if the child enjoyed music and found music pleasing or if there was a sensory avoidance to music or a specific type of music. Ideally, the practitioner can provide a variety of instruments for the child to choose from and use.

Instructions

1) The child chooses several music instruments and labels each one a different feeling.
2) The child then plays each instrument the way they think the feeling would sound.
3) The child is then instructed to choose the instruments/feelings that they often have and play those feelings.
4) The child is instructed to play feelings that they have often very loudly and for a longer amount of time. If they have the feeling just a little, then they should play the emotion softly for a shorter amount of time.
5) The practitioner then gives various scenarios to the child and the child has to decide what feeling(s) they think they would have in the scenario and play the appropriate instrument(s). The practitioner should create

scenarios that are relevant to the experiences of the child. For example, when another child at school calls you a mean name.

Rationale

Autistic and other neurodivergent children may positively respond to music-based interventions. This play intervention uses music to help children and adolescents work on identifying feelings and understanding and expressing feelings without needing verbal language. The intervention works on several areas related to emotional regulation and can be simplified for younger children and made more complex for adolescents. The practitioner can process through with the child any feelings that are identified.

Complete the Story

Therapy Needs: Feeling identification and expression, regulation, and connection
Level: Child, adolescent
Materials: Paper, pencil
Modality: Individual, group and family

Introduction

Complete the Story helps children identify feelings, what is creating the feeling, and what to do when a feeling is being experienced. The Complete the Story templates can be general or individualized to the specific child, addressing real-life situations that the child may be struggling with.

Instructions

The practitioner writes several stories about children in different situations. The stories should be brief and deal with a situation that is similar to things that are happening in the child's life. Each story will end with the following statement that the child has to complete:

The child feels _____ because _____, so they will _____

Example story to complete

Johnny went outside for recess. He wanted to play on the swings, but the swings were full. Johnny feels _____ because _____, so he will _____ _____

Rationale

This play intervention helps children and adolescents work on identifying feelings, understanding and expressing feelings, recognizing feelings in others, and overall emotion management. The practitioner should observe any struggles the child may have in completing the story and provide help if needed.

Complete the story examples

Mark went outside to play Pokémon Go, but he could not get the internet to work. Mark feels _____ because _____ _____, so he will _____.

Sarah wants to play by herself but other kids keep coming up to her and bothering her. Sarah feels _____ because _____ _____, so she will _____.

Michael's parents just told him he is going to his favorite amusement park. Michael feels _____ because _____ _____, so he will _____.

Hannah's grandmother died and Hannah is going to the funeral. Hannah feels _____ because _____ _____, so she will _____.

Travis has to give a speech in front of his class at school. Travis feels _____ because _____ _____, so he will _____.

Lily just won a special award for the best art drawing. Lily feels _____ because _____ _____, so she will _____.

Mason wanted to play kickball but the others kids would not let him. Mason feels _____ because _____ _____, so he will _____

Avatar My Feelings

(Contributed by Fiona Hill, Registered Play Therapist™)

Therapy Needs: Affect assessment, feeling identification
Level: Child, adolescent
Materials: Electronic device used for Telehealth, HIPAA compliant Zoom/Google Meet account (if using tablet for Telehealth the app version of Zoom or Google Meet will need to be downloaded on the device) enabled function to utilize avatar filters on the video platform
Modality: Individual, group

Introduction

Feeling identification can be difficult to navigate, both internally and through interactions with others. The use of play makes this endeavor fun, engaging and feel less overwhelming. Incorporating the use of digital tools has the potential to further encompass the child's world; therefore, creating a sense of felt safety and connection within the therapeutic relationship. One of the easiest and most accessible ways to incorporate digital tools in a virtual play therapy session is to use existing resources, such as features included within the Telehealth platform.

Instructions

1) When using or introducing any technique or intervention, two key components to rely on for guidance in determining its appropriateness are the child's interests and the existing therapeutic relationship. These two factors can help determine how, when, and even if the intervention is introduced in session.
2) Depending on the client and therapeutic relationship, the avatar may be able to 'just pop in' without warning. For some clients it may be necessary for the clinician to ask permission before turning on the filter in session. A fun way to discover which avatar the client is most drawn to is a type of show-and-tell with each avatar and inquire about the favorite, least favorite, etc.
3) When the avatar filter is enabled, it moves and pauses in sync with the user.
4) Zoom and Google Meet virtual platforms have a variety of avatars to choose from. While some fully embody the user, others allow space for the user's own face to be seen. There are benefits to both types in various situations.
5) Clinician as avatar: The clinician makes different facial expressions and uses the statement: 'When the cat (or other avatar) makes this face, it feels_____.' The client will then fill in the blank, indicating the emotion they associate with the facial expression.
6) Throughout the session, the clinician is tracking the client's interaction, expressions, and play; thus, helping the client to feel seen while simultaneously modeling identification of emotions

Rationale

Affect assessment gives the clinician insight into the client's ability to acknowledge, identify, and understand their own feelings as well as the feelings of others. The use of an avatar filter in this way allows the client to experience and identify feelings through a lens of distancing, much in the same way as using puppets. In contrast, avatar filters allow for the opportunity of embodiment while engaging in the therapeutic process. This intervention can easily be adapted for non-virtual sessions through the use of screenshots taken of various emotions and expressions.

Feeling 5

(Contributed by Danyale Weems, Registered Play Therapist Supervisor™)

Therapy Needs: Emotion regulation, feeling identification	
Level: Child, adolescent	
Materials: Intensity scale from 1–5; the numbers 1–5 (1 = low intensity (calmer) and 5 = high intensity (frustrated)) written out on large pieces of paper. It could also be created using colors or body templates with the numbers written on the body.	
Modality: Individual, family	

Introduction

Parents may struggle with understanding their neurodivergent child's intensity of feelings and how to help them manage their feelings. Neurodivergent children and adolescents may struggle to identify, express, and regulate their feelings. This play intervention helps the parents and child to understand feelings better. It also helps children and/or their parents to identify situations at various levels of intensity and support regulation.

Instructions

1) The practitioner and/or the parents identifies known situations (e.g. fire truck sirens, sibling yelling, noise in the cafeteria, being interrupted, tablet turning off, losing Wi-Fi, etc.) which typically creates a negative emotional reaction for the child. The identified situations are written on index cards or pieces of paper.

2) The practitioner displays a scale from 1–5 which can include color and emojis. The practitioner has pre-created the scale on a large piece of paper. The practitioner explains the 1–5 scale intensity and has the child/parents demonstrate with faces, noises, hand gestures, body movement etc. each of the levels. An alternative version would be to have the child and/or parents identify body sensations which connect to the levels (e.g. closed fists, pink cheeks, etc.).

3) The practitioner and/or parents reads a situation and then states to the child, 'This makes me feel ___.' The child takes the situation card and decides the intensity of the feeling by placing it on the large scale 1–5 intensity sheet.

4) If working with parents, they can have their own set to show where they think the child/adolescent's feeling intensity is at for a situation and this can be created into a game.

5) The practitioner and/or parents reflect and validate the child's feelings. At this point, for high-intensity reactions, a regulation activity can be practiced before moving to the next situation. Some activities might include deep breathing, bubble blowing, moving your body like a windmill, throwing and blowing cotton balls, playing a musical instrument, creating and flying a paper airplane, etc.

6) The process is continued until all the situations have been covered.

Rationale

This play intervention includes visual and kinesthetic learning. It provides an opportunity for the child to identify the intensity of their feelings and learn some ways to regulate their energy. Using this intervention can assist with regulation and sensory needs. When including the parent, this intervention can help create awareness about their child.

Feelings Pick-Up Sticks

Therapy Needs: Feeling identification and expression, regulation and connection
Level: Child, adolescent
Materials: Pick up sticks game, feeling/color sheet (in Appendix)
Modality: Individual, familygroup

Introduction

This play intervention utilizes the game Pick-Up Sticks to help increase feeling identification and emotional regulation in children and adolescents. Neurodivergent children may need help with a variety of knowledge points concerning their feeling and regulation system. This intervention provides the opportunity to individualize the activity to target any needs the child is experiencing.

Instructions

1) Using the game Pick-Up Sticks, the practitioner creates a sheet of paper with each Pick-Up Sticks color listed, and several feelings listed under each color.

2) The practitioner and child play a game of Pick-Up Sticks following the typical Pick-Up Sticks rules. It is important to note that some children will have trouble picking up some of the sticks without moving them. The practitioner should be lenient on this rule in the game, as the point is for the child to acquire a stick so they can share about a feeling.

3) When the practitioner or child picks up a stick of a certain color, they must look at the paper and pick one of the feelings listed under that color to share about a time they felt that way, act out the feeling, or define the feeling.

4) Play continues until all the sticks have been collected.

Rationale

This play intervention helps children and adolescents work on identifying feelings and understanding and expressing feelings through a popular game format. The practitioner can develop feeling/color sheets that address specific emotions that the practitioner believes the child may be struggling in identifying and expressing. Parents can be taught how to play this intervention, given a feelings sheet, and encouraged to purchase a Pick-Up Sticks game (they come in various sizes and are usually inexpensive). The game can be played several times and the feelings sheet can be changed as needed to work on new or more complex emotions. Parents can also create their own feelings sheets at home as needed.

Feelings Beach Ball

Therapy Needs: Feeling identification and expression, regulation, and connection
Level: Child, adolescent
Materials: Beach ball, black Sharpie pen
Modality: Individual, family, group

Introduction

Feelings Beach Ball provides an engaging and fun way for children and adolescents to work on a variety of feeling and regulation components. It is also an easy intervention for children and adolescents to take home and play with their family members. The practitioner can complete/design a beach ball prior to the child attending their session, individualizing the ball with specific feelings the child may need to address, or the practitioner and child can work together to create a feelings beach ball during the session.

Instructions

1) The practitioner blows up a beach ball and instructs the child that they are going to write feeling words all over the ball (the practitioner could create a beach ball with feelings on it prior to the child's session).
2) The child should think of as many feelings as they can, and the practitioner can add feelings to fill up the beach ball (the practitioner will want to make sure that feelings are included that the child needs to explore). A list of feelings is provided in the Appendix.
3) Once the ball is complete, the practitioner and child toss the ball back and forth. When someone catches the ball, whichever feeling is closest to the person's right thumb is the feeling they select and then share what makes them feel that way. Instead of sharing, they could act out the feeling while the other person tries to guess what it is.
4) If someone's thumb lands on a feeling that has already been done, they should choose the next feeling that is closest to their thumb.

5) An additional playful element would be to select different ways to toss the beach ball as it is passed back and forth such as, 'This time let's hit it to each other with our heads.'
6) Play continues until all the feelings are covered or the practitioner and child no longer want to play.

Rationale

This play intervention helps children and adolescents work on identifying feelings, understanding and expressing feelings, and understanding feelings in others. If the beach ball was individualized for the child, the child can take the beach ball home, and the practitioner can teach this intervention to parents to periodically play at home with their child. The child's feelings may change day-to-day and the level that the child is feeling will also change from day-to-day. Completing this technique periodically at home will help the child learn how feelings can change and how much a person feels a particular feeling can fluctuate, depending on the situation.

LEGO® Feeling House

Therapy Needs: Feeling identification and expression, regulation, and connection
Level: Child, adolescent
Materials: LEGO® bricks
Modality: Individual, group

Introduction

Several studies have supported the benefits of using LEGO® bricks with Autistic and other neurodivergent children and adolescents. This play intervention utilizes LEGO® play to work on increasing feeling identification and emotional regulation. The practitioner will ideally have a variety of LEGO® bricks for the child to access.

Instructions

1) The child is provided LEGO® bricks and instructed to build a house, a building of some type, or a car. The child can also build an abstract object if they would prefer.
2) The child is instructed that they will use different colors in their build and each color will represent a feeling.
3) The child should choose feelings that they experience often (the practitioner can also give the child a specific situation or person to identify feelings about such as school or their parents).

4) Once the child has constructed their object, the child goes through the colors and talks about each feeling and what causes them to have that feeling.
5) The practitioner may also inquire if the placement of the LEGO® bricks has any significance for the child.
6) The practitioner may also want to create a feelings house as well and role-model identifying and sharing feelings.

Rationale

LEGO® bricks are not only naturally inviting for a child (often a play preference) but can also provide a positive sensory and regulating experience. This play intervention helps children and adolescents work on identifying feelings and understanding and expressing feelings. The practitioner can teach this technique to parents to do periodically at home with their child. A child's feelings may change day-to-day and the level of feeling that a child is experiencing will also change from day-to-day. Completing this technique periodically at home can help the child develop better feeling identification and regulation ability. It can also help parents can gain a greater understating of what their child is feeling and helping their child to express their feelings.

Bean Bag Toss

Therapy Needs: Feeling identification and expression, regulation, and connection
Level: Child, adolescent
Materials: Bean bags, bucket
Modality: Individual, family

Introduction

This is a simple yet engaging intervention that helps children and adolescents work on a variety of feeling and regulation needs. The physical movement and challenge piece of the bean bag toss can also be good for helping children and adolescents learn to better regulate and accomplish a task. With Bean Bag Toss, the practitioner can individualize the intervention to address specific feeling/regulation needs that the child or adolescent needs to explore.

Instructions

1) Using some type of small bean bag, the practitioner will write a different feeling word on each bean bag (square, circle, or animal-shaped bean bags can be purchased through most toy stores – practitioners should purchase a type that can be written on with a Sharpie marker).

2) The child tries to throw the bean bags into a bucket that is set up some-where in the room.
3) For each bean bag the child gets in the bucket, the child will share the definition of the feeling or something that makes them feel that way.
4) The practitioner then takes a turn. The practitioner also defines the feeling or shares something that makes them feel that way.
5) The practitioner and child continue to take turns trying to get all the bean bags into the bucket and ultimately discussing all the feelings.
6) The intervention can be played several times with new information being shared about each feeling.

Rationale

Bean Bag Toss helps children and adolescents work on identifying, under-standing, and expressing feelings in a game completion format. This play intervention also involves a movement component and, after a couple of rounds, the practitioner can instruct the child that they are now going to play the game using their non-dominant hand to throw the bean bags. Another option would be trying to get the bean bags in the bucket by throwing them backwards over the head or some other silly move. The practitioner can teach this intervention to parents to do periodically at home with their child.

Feelings Spinner Game

Therapy Needs: Feeling identification and expression, regulation, and connection
Level: Child, adolescent
Materials: Color spinner (Figure 8.1 shows an example of a color spinner), paper, pencil
Modality: Individual, family, group

Introduction

Autistic and other neurodivergent children may struggle on some level with identifying feelings and emotional regulation ability. The Feelings Spinner Game is a simple, low prop intervention that can be constructed to work on any feeling or regulation component that a child or adolescent needs to explore. Children often enjoy using the spinner format and practitioners can involve children in the planning and set-up of the game.

Instructions

1) Using a color wheel spinner (typically purchased at an education supply store and can be purchased in bulk), the practitioner and child decide what feeling will go with each color on the wheel spinner and write the feelings down on a piece of paper, such as yellow = happy, red = mad, blue = worried, green = sad, etc.

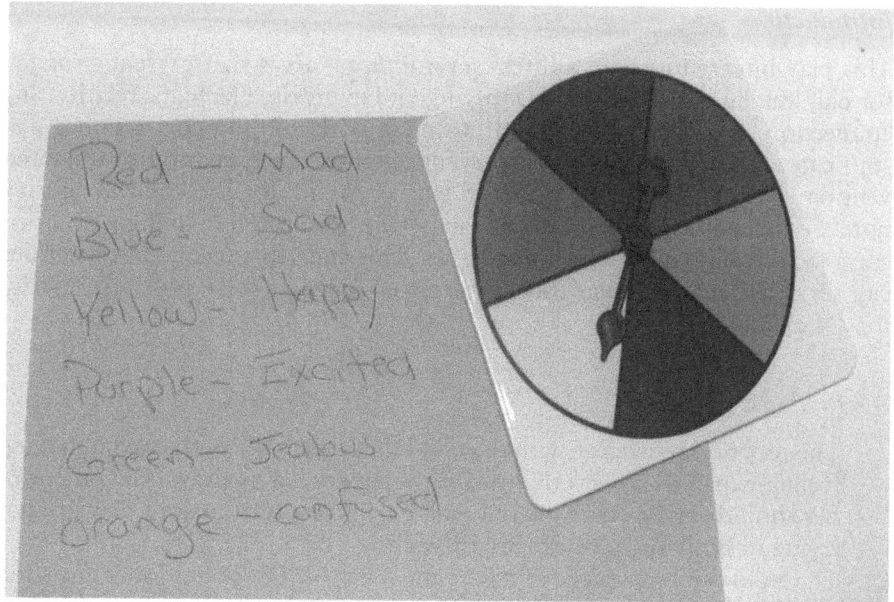

Figure 8.1 Feelings spinner game.

Robert Jason Grant

2) The practitioner and child then take turns spinning the spinner. When someone spins the spinner, whichever color the spinner lands on, the person has to act out the feeling or tell about a time they felt that way. The same feeling can be landed on several times with new information shared about that feeling. Play continues until the practitioner and child want to stop.

Rationale

Feelings Spinner Game helps children and adolescents work on identifying and understanding feelings and emotional regulation. Several different emotional regulation components can be addressed with this intervention. The practitioner can vary the spinner creation and game rules in any way they think may be more applicable to the child's therapy goals. The spinner can be sent home and parents taught how to play the game with their child.

Draw My Feelings Face

Therapy Needs: Feeling identification and expression, regulation, and connection	
Level: Child, adolescent	
Materials: Paper, pencil	
Modality: Individual, family, group	

Introduction

This play intervention can address several target areas that present struggles for children and adolescents. Identifying and expressing feelings, relationship connection, and social navigation (attuning with and noticing another person) can all be included in the intervention play. The execution of the intervention should be fun and silly and stay engaging for the child. Affirming note: Some neurodivergent children may be uncomfortable looking at a person's face and/or have alexithymia issues. This and other feeling interventions can serve as an assessment tool to better understand these possible descriptors of children.

Instructions

1) The practitioner shares with the child that they will be practicing making feeling expression faces that the other person has to draw. The practitioner should explain that the drawing part is just for fun, and they are not trying to draw the face exactly or well.
2) The child is given a piece of paper and a pencil. The practitioner goes first by making a feeling face for about three seconds. The face should be fun and exaggerated.
3) The child draws the feeling face the practitioner made and writes on the paper or says out loud the feeling word that they believe goes with the practitioner's face. The practitioner confirms if the child is correct. If the answer is not correct, the practitioner should make the face again and provide some hints.
4) The child goes next and makes a feeling face expression and the practitioner draws what they believe it is. The practitioner and child take turns back and forth with each one making a feeling face and the other drawing and labeling what they saw.
5) Play continues until the practitioner and child no longer want to play.

Rationale

This play intervention is designed to address therapy goals related to feeling identification, relationship development and social navigation. Some feelings will be difficult to display with a facial expression, or a facial expression might be appropriate for several different feelings. Some neurodivergent children may not recognize or 'read' facial expression very well. This provides a good opportunity for discussion on how to handle situations when it is difficult to understand a person's facial expressions.

Feelings Don't Break The Ice®

Therapy Needs: Feeling identification and expression, regulation, and connection
Level: Child

Materials: Don't Break The Ice boardgame by Hasbro, stickers
Modality: Individual, group, family

Introduction

Don't Break The Ice® is a popular boardgame that is naturally engaging for children. This intervention utilizes this game to help children differentiate between positive and negative feelings and identify what could create certain feelings. The typical game rules are followed with some additional feeling instructions.

Instructions

1) Using the Don't Break The Ice boardgame by Hasbro, the practitioner takes each of the 'ice' pieces and on the underside of each piece, puts a color sticker or a symbol sticker such as a star or heart.
2) There should be four different colors or symbols represented and a few of the 'ice' pieces left blank with no sticker on them (this is done prior to playing the game with any child).
3) The practitioner instructs the child that they are going to play Feelings Don't Break The Ice.
4) The practitioner shows the child the stickers on the ice pieces and the practitioner and child decide together which two colors/symbols of stickers will represent positive feelings and which two colors/symbols will represent negative feelings. For example, the practitioner and child might decide that green and blue will be positive feelings and red and yellow will be negative feelings.
5) The normal Don't Break The Ice rules are observed with an additional rule; once an ice piece is knocked out, if it has a sticker on the underside, the person who knocked that piece out has to identify a positive or negative feeling (depending on the color) and talk about something that has made them feel that way.
6) Play continues as normal in Don't Break The Ice rules. The practitioner and child can replay the game several times.

Rationale

This play intervention helps children work on increasing feeling identification and expression. It also provides relationship development and social navigation (turn-taking, playing a game together, winning and losing). The focus is on helping children identify positive and negative feelings and learning how to express those feelings. Parents can be encouraged to purchase the game and taught to play this intervention at home with their child. Practitioners should also consider that the colored stickers can be used to represent other areas besides feelings, such as social questions, coping skills, or regulation motor movements.

Happy Me, Sad Me

Therapy Needs: Feeling identification and expression, regulation, and connection
Level: Child, adolescent
Materials: Paper, pencil
Modality: Individual, group

Introduction

This play intervention is simple yet engaging for children and adolescents and presents a strong visual representation of the child's feelings and connecting their feelings to situations. Happy and sad are the primary focus, but other feelings can be incorporated such as mad me, brave me, scared me, worried me, excited me, or calm me. Practitioners can choose feelings that the child needs to explore and repeat this intervention using different feelings each time.

Instructions

1) The practitioner instructs the child to draw a line down the middle of a piece of paper. On one side of the paper the child will draw a happy self and on the other side a sad self. Words or happy and sad face stickers can be used to title each side.
2) Underneath the happy self, the child will write all the things they can think of that make them feel happy. Underneath the sad self, the child will write all the things they can think of that make them feel sad. These can be current things or past things, there are no limits.
3) If the child is struggling to identify things that make them feel happy and sad, the practitioner can help the child by asking them questions such as, 'What is your favorite class in school?', 'What feelings do you have when you are in that class?', 'What is something you don't like to do?', 'What feelings do you have when you have to do that thing?'
4) Once the lists are complete, the practitioner and child go through both lists, talking about each thing the child has identified.
5) At this point, the child could complete another sheet with two different feelings.

Rationale

The Happy Me, Sad Me play intervention can help children work on increasing feelings identification and expression. The happy/sad sheet provides a strong visual reminder that the child can take home and reference. Various feelings can be used to complete this intervention, but there should always be a positive emotion that contrasts with a negative emotion. Parents can be taught to complete this intervention at home and encouraged to look for opportunities to play with their child, especially days or times when it may seem their child is experiencing some negative emotions.

Feelings Card Sort

Therapy Needs: Feeling identification and expression, regulation, relationships, and connection
Level: Adolescent
Materials: Several index cards, pen or pencil
Modality: Individual

Introduction

Adolescents can have a challenging time communicating about their feelings especially in regard to the relationships in their lives. Feelings Card Sort helps adolescents accurately identify and discriminate between feelings that they may be experiencing specifically related to various family member relationships.

Instructions

1) The practitioner explains that the adolescent will be using index cards to help identify the various feelings that they may have regarding different relationships in their life.
2) The adolescent writes as many feelings as they can think of on index cards (one feeling per index card). The practitioner can also add feelings/ index cards so there is a variety of feelings represented on the index cards.
3) The adolescent then makes an index card for each family member with the family member's name written on the card.
4) The practitioner takes the family member cards and, one at a time, lays down a family member card and the adolescent has to choose from the feeling index cards, feelings they have for that family member and then lays down those feeling cards with the family member card.
5) The practitioner and adolescent then discuss why they chose those feelings about that family member.
6) The practitioner and adolescent go through this process for each family member card.
7) An alternate version can be to have the practitioner lay down a family member card and the adolescent must choose feeling index cards that represent feelings that the adolescent thinks that family member feels about them. The practitioner and adolescent then discuss why they believe that family member would have those feelings.

Rationale

The Feelings Card Sort intervention helps adolescents work on identifying feelings, understanding and expressing feelings, and exploring family relationships. The card sort game can be expanded beyond family member relationships and include other people in the adolescent's life such as friends, teachers, doctors, etc.

Feelings Quiz

Therapy Needs: Feeling identification and expression, regulation, social engagement, and connection
Level: Child, adolescent
Materials: Paper, pencil
Modality: Individual, group

Introduction

This play intervention is implemented in a game format and helps children and adolescents who may be struggling with identifying and connecting to feelings. The quiz format provides a fun and engaging way for children to think about feelings and to try and name as many feelings as they can. Practitioners should make the feelings quiz lively, dramatic, and fun.

Instructions

1) The practitioner instructs the child or adolescent that they are going to complete a feelings quiz.
2) The practitioner should announce this in a grandiose way and try to keep the process light, not serious like a true formal quiz, and not competitive.
3) The child has to name a certain number of feelings. The number depends on the age and developmental level of the child. The practitioner should try to pick a number that would be challenging yet attainable for the child. It is important that the child be successful in identifying the feelings.
4) The child begins to name off feelings and the practitioner writes them down to keep track of what has been said and when the number has been reached.
5) The practitioner can provide hints to help the child identify feelings. An example hint would be to instruct the child to think about a specific place or situation like school or being on vacation and what feelings they noticed in that place or situation.
6) Once the child has identified the number required, the practitioner can provide a small prize such as a ribbon, sticker, or piece of candy. The prize is optional but can be fun and celebratory for the child.

Rationale

This play intervention helps children and adolescents work on identifying feelings. This intervention can usually be done quickly and does not require the whole session time so it can be paired with other interventions. This intervention can also be done periodically (a 'pop' feelings quiz) throughout working with the child to see if they can progress in the number of feelings they can identify. The practitioner can chart progress as the child increases in their ability to identify more feelings without needing any hints. The Feelings Quiz can serve as an informal quantitative measure that evaluates the child's ability to increase feeling identification.

Write a Feelings Story

Therapy Needs: Feeling identification and expression, regulation, and connection
Level: Child, adolescent
Materials: Paper, pencil
Modality: Individual, familygroup

Introduction

Neurodivergent children may need help exploring feelings, especially conceptualizing feelings. This play intervention helps children more fully conceptualize feelings. The child works on identifying feelings, understanding what may be creating a certain feeling, and recognizing feelings in others. A story format is used so multiple feelings stories can be created to present various feelings and situations.

Instructions

1) The practitioner has the child or adolescent complete a short story that has pre-placed emotion words. The child can write whatever story they want with the goal to match up to the preplaced feeling words. The therapist should have the templates ready to go before the child's session.

Example template

_____ happy _____
_____
_____ sad _____ shy _____
_____ loved _____
_____ angry _____
_____ excited _____ worried _____
_____

2) Once the child has completed the story, they read the story to the practitioner. The practitioner can process with the child the story that they created. The practitioner can assist younger children and children who cannot, or do not want to, write with the completing of the story.
3) Several template examples are provided in the appendix.

Rationale

The conceptualization of feelings can be difficult for some children and requires practice to improve. This play intervention helps children and adolescents work on identifying and understanding emotions through a story creation format. Story templates are included in the Appendix, but practitioners can easily create their own. Practitioners should let children know that the lines in the template are an approximate as some children may need more room to write out their story between pre-placed feelings. Practitioners can also allow children to create their own templates if they desire.

Feeling Fortune Tellers

Therapy Needs: Feeling identification and expression, regulation, engagement, and connection
Level: Child, adolescent
Materials: Paper, markers
Modality: Individual, family, group

Introduction

Neurodivergent children may need to explore multiple components related to feeling identification and regulation. The Feeling Fortune Tellers intervention provides the opportunity to practice several different areas related to feelings. The practitioner can make the instructions to focus on any area of feeling identification, expression, or regulation they would like the child to practice such as, sharing about a time you felt that way, show how you would feel, act out the feeling, tell about a time you noticed someone else feeling this feeling, define the feeling, or how you could express or regulate that feeling. Children typically enjoy the construction, movement, and game format of the fortune tellers and usually desire creating multiple fortune tellers.

Instructions

1) The practitioner explains to the child that they will be creating a paper feeling fortune teller (instructions for completion can be found online).
2) Fortune tellers should have numbers on the outside, colors on the inside, and feeling words placed on the tab on the other side of the colors.

3) After the fortune teller has been created, the practitioner and child can take turns playing the game.
4) The basic process of the game is as follows: The practitioner holds the fortune teller in their fingers. The child chooses a number, and the practitioner moves the fortune teller back and forth the number of times for the number that the child chose. The practitioner opens up the fortune teller and the child selects a color. The practitioner lifts the flap for that color, which reveals a feeling. The child has to follow whatever instruction has been decided about what to do with the feeling word.
5) The practitioner and child take turns back and forth with the fortune teller and play continues until they no longer want to play.

Rationale

This play intervention can assist with feeling identification, expression of feelings, and a variety of regulation needs. The fortune tellers can be made in different sizes and different colors using construction paper. The practitioner and child can play the fortune teller game several times. The child can take their fortune tellers home and play with other family members. Parents can be encouraged to make additional feeling fortune tellers at home with their child. The instructions for creating and playing fortune tellers can be easily accessed online with picture and video examples.

Feelings Puzzle

Therapy Needs: Feeling identification and expression, regulation, and connection
Level: Child, adolescent
Materials: Blank puzzle (6–9 pieces), markers
Modality: Individual, family, group

Introduction

Autistic and other neurodivergent children can be strong visual learners. This play intervention provides a strong visual representation of different feelings that children can remember and helps them identify feelings that they may experience regularly. The tactile and puzzle completion component also provides a sense of engagement, order, and creation for the child.

Instructions

1) The practitioner tells the child they will be using a blank puzzle to create a puzzle focused on feelings.
2) The practitioner instructs the child to write a different feeling word on the back side of each puzzle piece of a blank puzzle.

3) The practitioner may have to help the child think of different feelings and should try to include negative feelings that the child may need to explore.
4) On the front side of the puzzle, the child can decorate the puzzle however they want.
5) Once the puzzle has been completed, the puzzle is taken apart and the practitioner and child put the puzzle back together. Each time a piece of the puzzle is connected, the child has to share when they felt that feeling (written on the back side of the puzzle piece) or act out what the feeling would look like.

Rationale

The Feelings Puzzle helps children and adolescents work on identifying feelings and understanding and expressing feelings through a visual creation of a puzzle. The puzzle pieces provide a strong visual representation of feelings for the child and the actions of taking apart and putting the puzzle back together help to strengthen the child's familiarity with the targeted feelings. Children should take their puzzles home and put them together with their parents and work with their parents on sharing and identifying feelings. Parents and children can also make new puzzles with different feeling words. Blank puzzles come in several sizes and various numbers of pieces. A good basic size for children is a small puzzle with 6–9 pieces. Puzzles with more pieces might be selected for adolescents. Blank puzzles can be ordered online from several retailers.

Paper Feelings Balloons

Therapy Needs: Feeling identification and expression, regulation, and connection
Level: Child, adolescent
Materials: Paper, markers, pencil, balloons
Modality: Individual

Introduction

The Paper Feelings Balloons intervention is a fun and engaging way to help children think about different situations and the feelings that they may experience in each situation. Children are often able to identify more feelings by thinking of specific situations, environments, or people and recognizing feelings they have regarding specific qualifiers.

Instructions

1) The child is instructed to draw one large balloon in the corner of a piece of paper.

2) The child is instructed to write as many feelings as they can think of inside the large balloon. This is the master balloon the child will be referring to.
3) The child is then instructed to draw four smaller balloons on the paper; each balloon should be a different color.
4) The practitioner takes the paper and labels one of the smaller balloons a subject such as school. The child then writes all the feelings that they can think of that they feel about school on that balloon.
5) The child can reference their master balloon. If they think of a feeling that was not written on the master balloon, then they write that feeling in both the school balloon and the master balloon.
6) When the child is finished with the school balloon, they can get a real balloon that they can keep and take home.
7) This process is repeated for the other three balloons, with the practitioner labeling each one with a different subject and the child identifying feelings that they have regarding that subject.
8) Some subject ideas might include school, home, mom, dad, my siblings, music class, band, the doctor's office, playing video games etc.
9) The practitioner should try to pick subjects that will produce a wide variety of feelings for the child. When all the balloons have been completed, the practitioner and child can discuss all the feelings that the child identified. An example paper feelings balloons is provided in Figure 8.2.

Rationale

This play intervention helps children and adolescents work on identifying feelings and understanding and expressing feelings. It also helps children understand that they can have more than one feeling about a subject and some of those feelings might be a mix of both positive and negative feelings. Children are typically able to identify more feelings by having them consider specific situations and the feelings they have in that situation. Children can take this intervention home and complete more feelings balloons with their parents.

Feeling List Stop Game

Therapy Needs: Feeling identification and expression, regulation, and connection
Level: Child, adolescent
Materials: Paper, pencil
Modality: Individual

Introduction

The Feeling List Stop Game is a simple but effective way for children and adolescents to think about feelings, share what makes them feel certain ways,

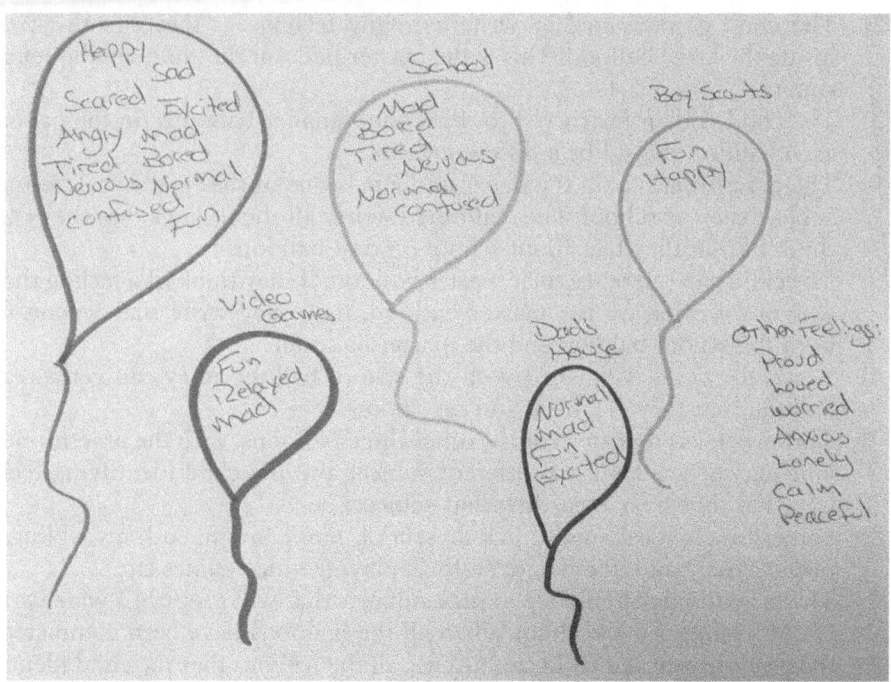

Figure 8.2 Paper feelings balloons.

Robert Jason Grant

and communicate what they can do to help themselves feel more regulated when they are experiencing a negative feeling.

Instructions

1) The child is instructed to make a list of 12 feelings (the child can look at a feelings chart or the feelings list provided in the Appendix of this book to help them identify the feelings).
2) The child writes the feelings on a piece of paper, down the side, numbered 1–12 (a worksheet example is provided in the Appendix).
3) Once the child has completed the list, the practitioner takes the list and instructs the child that the practitioner is going to run their finger up and down the list without looking at the list and when the child says stop, the practitioner will stop and whatever feeling the practitioner's finger is on, the child has to share when they felt that way, and if it is a negative feeling, the child has to share what they could do to help them feel better.
4) The practitioner may have to help the child, depending on the child's age and developmental level. When discussing a negative feeling, the practitioner and child can also role-play through any identified strategies for coping better or regulating through the negative emotion.

5) The practitioner and child can also switch roles and the practitioner can share their feelings and role-model for the child how to discuss feelings and ideas for handling negative feelings.
6) Play continues until all feelings have been chosen or until the practitioner and child no longer want to play.

Rationale

The Feeling Stop List Game helps children and adolescents work on identifying feelings and understanding and expressing feelings. This play intervention can be played repeatedly, creating new lists with new feelings. Variations can also be added like acting out the feeling. Children often enjoy switching roles with the practitioner and running their finger up and down the list, with the practitioner sharing their feelings. Parents can be taught this intervention to play at home and encouraged to play with their child regularly.

Anxiety Mometer

Therapy Needs: Feeling identification and expression, regulation, and connection	
Level: Child, adolescent	
Materials: Paper, markers	
Modality: Individual, family, group	

Introduction

Autistic and other neurodivergent children and adolescents can sometimes have difficulty differentiating between levels of dysregulation or anxiety. This play intervention helps children and adolescents learn to identify different levels of dysregulation and situations or triggers that create levels of anxiety.

Instructions

1) The practitioner and/or child draw a thermometer outline on a piece of paper (a thermometer template could also be used).
2) The practitioner and child decide on different situations to place on the thermometer, from situations that create no anxiety for the child placed at the bottom of the thermometer and progressively moving up the thermometer, with different situations that increasingly create more anxiety or dysregulation for the child.
3) The practitioner and child then review all the situations and talk about interventions that the child can do at each level to help them regulate.
4) The practitioner can write on the paper beside the thermometer different intervention ideas for the child to implement when they are at different levels on the thermometer. The practitioner and child can then role-play

through several situations that create anxiety and practice implementing an intervention to help decrease the anxiety and dysregulation.

5) This is an intervention that can be completed regularly in other sessions to continue the process of identifying anxiety and dysregulation triggers, and developing regulation strategies.

Rationale

This play intervention helps children and adolescents work on decreasing anxiety and dysregulation. It provides the opportunity for children and adolescents to learn to identify when they are beginning to feel dysregulated and attend to the dysregulation before it amplifies. The practitioner should have a clear understanding of different situations that create different levels of anxiety for the child. Practitioners may want to consult with the child's parents before completing this intervention. Children should keep the anxiety mometer posted at home to reference. Parents can be taught this intervention and encouraged to implement the intervention at home. Parents can also be encouraged to direct their child to their anxiety mometer when they notice their child becoming dysregulated and help their child implement a regulation strategy through a co-regulation process.

9 Regulation Interventions

Create and Contain aka Take Your Power Back

(Contributed by Tony Vallance, Clinical Play Therapist)

Therapy Needs: Regulation, anxiety reduction, power and control issues
Level: Adolescent (not recommended for individuals with any history of psychosis or reality perception issues)
Materials: Meta Quest 2 virtual reality headset, laptop, minimum 6 x 6ft space, 6 degrees of freedom VR is recommended for ages 12 and up, pencils and paper for initial sketching.
Modality: Individual

Introduction

This externalization-based intervention leverages the immersive quality of virtual reality (VR) in a safe, expressive, and empowering way. It uses a creative program called Tilt Brush which enables participants to draw using a broad range of tools (from virtual paint brushes to painting with rainbows, fire and light) in three dimensions in the space around them. In this environment in VR, they can create a representation of a particular challenge or frustration (identified first in talk based or hand drawn sketching) and then shrink it down to be very small before them. Then they may create a distancing or containment model or design around the threat/challenge/frustration. Pre- and post-reflections can be done about how they feel about the creation before containing it and after.

Instructions

1) The adolescent is instructed to think about a particular frustration, challenge, or threat that they have to deal with and to sketch it on paper.
2) Next, they put the Meta Quest 2 headset on (Tilt Brush should have already been loaded up and casting set so the practitioner can see on their

DOI: 10.4324/9781003398691-9

computer/laptop what the adolescent can see; this enables the practitioner to using tracking behaviors whilst they are in VR).
3) The adolescent draws their sketch in Tilt Brush.
4) After the adolescent has drawn a model/representation of their object of frustration, they are shown how to use the scale tool to reduce the model size until it is very small in front of them.
5) Now they are instructed to create a way to contain that frustration. If using a more directive approach, the practitioner may suggest creating bars like a jail around the object.
6) The practitioner should reflect on how the adolescent feels to see the size of their frustration, challenge, or threat reduced and contained.

Rationale

Externalization using software such as Tilt Brush in VR can be very powerful in helping a participant to create a representation of their frustration, challenge, or threat and control its scale, severity, and spread. Often when feeling voiceless, choiceless, and disempowered, creating an immersive representation of the cause/s of those feelings and then shrinking and containing them can be extremely empowering when it comes to perception of those challenges outside of the therapeutic space.

Make a Dragon Egg

(Contributed by Jessamy Whitsitt, Play and Family Therapist)

Therapy Needs: Regulation, relationship, sensory needs, anxiety reduction, executive functioning needs, and connection
Level: Child, adolescent
Materials: Baking soda, flour (can use gluten-free flour), water, food coloring or paint, vinegar, thick paper plate or disposable plastic plate
Modality: Individual, family, group

Introduction

Meeting a child where they are at is key to relationship building in the therapeutic process. Getting creative and messy while working together can grow your connection by leaps and bounds. When working with neurodivergent children, incorporating their special interest into the intervention brings additional buy-in, as it adds an extra level of much needed attunement that they may not receive in their day-to-day lives. This play intervention helps with regulation and executive functioning as it involves following simple, straightforward directions to get the right mix to create the egg to surround the small plastic toy. (You can use any item that makes sense for the client; for this example a dragon is used.) Sensory integration occurs as the client mixes the creation with tools and/or their hands, smells the mixture and sees things as it starts to take shape. Anxiety reduction occurs when the connection is made with a trusted adult that sees the client and values their special interest in dragons, dinosaurs, fairies, etc. Additional skills of self-advocacy can occur if the client asks for help in forming the egg, as well as frustration tolerance if the dragon keeps popping its head out and needs to be covered in a different way to make sure it gets fully immersed in the mixture.

Instructions

1) The practitioner instructs the client to pour about 1 cup of baking soda and 2 spoons of flour onto the plate and mix in about ¼ cup of water until they get a dough-type texture.
2) As it comes together, they can start forming an egg-shape ball.
3) Once it feels like a good texture that will come together, split it in half and stick a small plastic toy in middle (dragon, dinosaur, whatever the child likes).
4) Stick each half over the toy and press firmly to shape it over toy. It will be a bit crumbly and may fall off in parts. If more water is needed, the child can dip their fingers in the water to add additional moisture. If additional mixture is needed, make a little more to the side to add on to ensure the item is fully coated.
5) Once firmly coated, dab drops of food coloring or paint to speckle the egg in any design.
6) Let the egg fully dry for several hours or overnight before attempting to hatch.
7) The child can take the egg home and hatch it in a bin or sink using 1 cup of vinegar to pour over the egg. The egg will bubble and begin to hatch and then whatever tools a parent will allow can be used to produce the small toy inside. If the egg is kept at the therapy office, have vinegar on hand for the next session to do the hatching process with client.

Rationale

This play intervention can achieve a variety of goals, depending on the child and how the practitioner approaches the implementation. The relationship building and sensory aspects of this intervention can help with anxiety reduction. Following basic instructions to get the egg to take shape helps with executive functioning. Integrating the senses occurs as the client mixes the dough by hand, smells the concoction, and see the bright colors as they speckle their egg. When they hatch their egg, additional benefits of stimulating their senses using vinegar to help hatch the egg occurs, as well as the motor skills used to chip away at the egg with playdough tools or other kitchen utensils. Getting messy can be fun for some neurodivergent children and reduce anxiety, while for others it can build tolerance in doing something they want to do but not loving the way it feels on their hands.

Volcano and Rain

Therapy Needs: Regulation, feeling identification and expression
Level: Child, adolescent
Materials: Paper, markers
Modality: Individual, group

Introduction

Volcano and rain is a play intervention that presents a strong visual for helping children and adolescents identify what creates anxiety or dysregulation in their life and ways to regulate and modulate their emotions. This intervention involves drawing and a more expressive process which may be a play preference for some children.

Instructions

1) The practitioner explains to the child that they are going to draw a picture of a volcano on the bottom side of a piece of paper and on the top side, they are going to draw some clouds and some large rain drops.
2) The practitioner instructs the child to write on the volcano anything they can think of that creates anxiety, dysregulation, or anger for them.
3) In the rain drops, the child will write anything they can think of that helps them calm down or feel regulated when they are feeling upset.
4) The practitioner may need to assist the child in identifying both things that upset them and things that help them regulate.
5) Once the volcano and rain have been created, the practitioner and child discuss all the things that upset the child and practice all the regulating/calming strategies that have been identified. Figure 9.1 provides a volcano and rain example.

Rationale

This play intervention helps children and adolescents work on decreasing dysregulation and identifying and expressing feelings. This intervention can be used to target a specific emotion such as worry or anger or a more general concept such as feeling dysregulated. The drawing can be taken home, and the child can hang it up somewhere visible where they can reference their drawing when they are feeling upset.

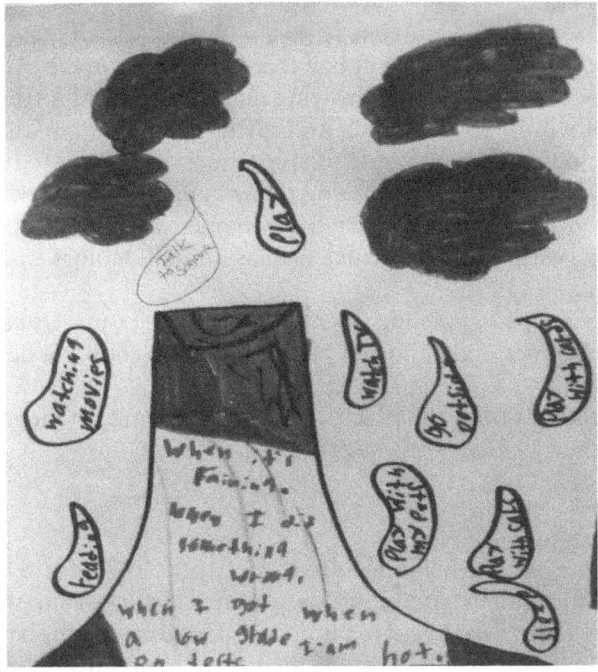

Figure 9.1 Volcano and Rain Example (child writing on the volcano things that make them angry and in the rain drops things that help them feel regulated).

Robert Jason Grant

Brain Ball

Therapy Needs: Regulation, executive functioning needs, social navigation (game play)
Level: Child, adolescent
Materials: Soft ball
Modality: Individual, group

Introduction

Neurodivergent children can become dysregulated and that dysregulation can often lead to an emotion and/or behavior meltdown. Helping children learn 're-set' brain activities to get their thoughts off their dysregulation and activate their whole brain can be helpful in reducing dysregulation. Brain Ball is a fun and engaging way to activate the whole brain and help children 're-set' from their dysregulation.

Instructions

1) The practitioner selects a soft ball that will be used in the play and instructs the client that they will be throwing the ball back and forth to each other.
2) The ball will be thrown back and forth in a rhythm, with the ball being held no longer than a couple of seconds.
3) At the same time the ball is being thrown, in rhythm (back and forth), the practitioner and child must call out names of things from a pre-chosen category (without any repeats) such as animals, colors, sports, emotions, fruits, etc.
4) The play keeps happening until someone messes up. Once this happens, the practitioner and child can begin again and choose a new topic if they want.
5) Play continues until the practitioner and child are no longer interested in playing.

Rationale

This play intervention helps children to re-focus off their dysregulation or anxiety and focus their attention in a way that activates the whole brain. (It is important that the category naming is paired with the ball throwing in order to activate the whole brain.) This helps children to regulate, calm, and re-set their emotions and thinking. This intervention should be played several times until the child begins to feel more regulated and less anxious.

Balloon Relay

Therapy Needs: Regulation, anxiety reduction, executive functioning needs
Level: Child and adolescent
Materials: Balloon
Modality: Individual, family, group

Introduction

Balloon Relay incorporates a game format to help address regulation needs. The intervention instructions require children to incorporate whole-brain movements with concentration and focus. The goal is to help children who are feeling dysregulated to regulate, calm, and re-set their anxious feelings and thoughts.

Instructions

1) The practitioner and child blow up two balloons.
2) The practitioner gives the instructions to the child that they each will have a balloon and they are going to go across the room and back, hitting the balloon in the air in a certain way.

3) The practitioner and child might start with moving across the room hitting their balloons in the air using only their pinky finger.
4) Once they have gone across the room and back, they switch to another way to hit the balloon such as with their heads only.
5) The practitioner and child hit their balloons across the room and back several times incorporating several different ways. Some other examples include knee, hands, nose, feet, hopping on one foot, etc.
6) Play continues until the practitioner and child no longer want to play.

Rationale

This play intervention helps children and adolescents work on decreasing dysregulation and learning a strategy to help decrease anxiety. This intervention activates the child's whole brain through specific movements and concentration tasks. Balloon Relay should be played several times in a row, incorporating several different ways to hit the balloon across the room. This intervention can also be paired with other regulation interventions.

Roll of the Dice

Therapy Needs: Regulation	
Level: Child, adolescent	
Materials: Dice, paper, pencil	
Modality: Individual, family, group	

Introduction

The Roll of the Dice intervention gives the practitioner the ability to practice specific regulation strategies that the child or adolescent is struggling with and needs to improve upon. The dice provides a fun way for the child to engage and participate in practicing regulation tools. The child can participate in thinking about and deciding what regulation tools they believe are helpful to their system.

Instructions

1) The practitioner explains to the child that they are going to play a game and practice some regulation strategies.
2) The practitioner and child write down on a piece of paper six regulation tools and number them 1 through 6. The practitioner should let the child try to think of some regulation strategies they believe are helpful and then the practitioner can complete the list with additional ideas.
3) The child will then roll the dice and practice the matching numbered strategy.

4) After the child has practiced that strategy, they will roll the dice again and try to get a different number to practice.
5) This will continue until all six regulation tools have been chosen and practiced.
6) The practitioner role-plays and practices each strategy with the child. After all six strategies have been practiced, the practitioner and child can play the game again with the same tools or create six new regulation tools
7) The practitioner should try to make the game fun and engaging for the child. The practitioner can incorporate props such as hats, masks, toys, etc. to try to make the practice more enjoyable.

Rationale

This play intervention helps children and adolescents work on addressing regulation needs. This intervention allows the practitioner and child to explore what regulation tools would be helpful for the child. In this way, the intervention also serves as an assessment to discover more about the child's regulation system. Parents can be taught how to do this intervention at home and encouraged to play with the entire family.

Prevention Role-Play

Therapy Needs: Regulation, feeling identification, anxiety reduction	
Level: Child, adolescent	
Materials: None	
Modality: Individual	

Introduction

Autistic and other neurodivergent children may find themselves in specific situations or events that create a great deal of anxiety and dysregulation for them. Parents often have a difficult time getting their children to participate in dysregulating events, such as getting their hair cut or going to the dentist. Prevention role-play can help children and adolescents reduce anxiety levels, gain confidence, and regulate through specific scenarios and events that are typically troublesome for them.

Instructions

1) The practitioner should begin by identifying what specific situation(s) or event(s) a child is struggling with.
2) More than likely this can be identified by the parents. For example, the parents may identify that going to the doctor is a struggle. The child has

had several meltdowns and often the parents cannot get the child to go into the doctor's office.

3) The practitioner would gather as much information from the parents as possible about going to the doctor, such as the doctor's name, what the office is like, what the usual procedures are, and what the child's specific reactions and behavior are like.

4) The practitioner then meets with the child and role-plays the situation with the child in a fun, engaging, and somewhat exaggerated way.

5) The practitioner may begin by using puppets or people figures or use themselves to play the roles of the child and the doctor and the parent.

6) The practitioner should use props such as dress-up clothes and masks to make the role-play fun, active, and playful, exaggerating all the reactions. The practitioner will likely use a whole variety of props from the playroom.

7) The practitioner will ask the child to participate in the role-play and let the child participate at the level they are comfortable with.

8) The practitioner will encourage the child to take on more and more of the role-play until the child is fully participating and playing themself and going through the role-play.

9) When the role-play, depicting the actual events, has been played several times, the practitioner will introduce playing the role-play with a positive outcome where the child uses coping/regulation tools and goes to the doctor without having a meltdown or getting upset.

10) The practitioner and child will then play through the new role-play several times until the end of the session.

11) The role-play may be repeated in the next session and several more sessions until the child can successfully participate in going to the doctor. It is most helpful to begin this intervention a few sessions prior to the event the child will be participating in.

Rationale

Prevention role-play is designed to help children practice regulation to help them participate in challenging situations or events that create a great deal of anxiety or dysregulation. This intervention also helps children become desensitized to the troubling situation or event. The role-play should be played many times to help the child decrease anxiety regarding the troubling event. The practitioner will want to gain feedback from the parents on how the child handled the situation after participating in the prevention role-play intervention. Parents can also role-play with their child at home. Parents will especially want to implement this intervention a few days prior to attending the targeted event.

Examples of typical dysregulating situations

Going to the doctor
Going to the dentist

Getting a haircut
Going to a grocery or department store
Going through a car wash
Attending school assemblies
Participating in school field trips
Going to fairs and carnivals
Going to jump houses and arcades
Attending family reunions
Attending a birthday party
Having relatives visit
Going on a vacation
Flying in an airplane
Going through airport security
Using a public restroom
Ordering food at a restaurant
Going to a theme park
Playing at a park
Going to a swimming pool

Feelings Field Trip

Therapy Needs: Regulation, feeling identification and expression	
Level: Child, adolescent	
Materials: Construction paper, markers	
Modality: Individual, group	

Introduction

Many neurodivergent children are strong visual learners. This play intervention provides a visual and kinesthetic learning/processing experience for addressing feelings and regulating the system. It also provides a tool that children can use at home to express negative or overwhelming emotions.

Instructions

1) The practitioner instructs the child to choose a color of construction paper that they associate with an anxious or worried feeling.
2) The practitioner explains to the child that they are going on a feelings field trip.
3) The practitioner instructs the child to write on the construction paper all the things that they can think of that make them feel anxious or worried. The practitioner can help the child by adding things to the list and verifying with the child that what the practitioner added is relevant for the child.

4) The practitioner and child read through the list making sure everything is listed that is relevant.
5) The practitioner instructs the child to rip the paper into pieces and think about getting rid of all the worried and anxious feelings while they are ripping up the paper.
6) The child gathers up all the ripped-up pieces, and the practitioner and child take their 'field trip' to an outside trash can, throwing all the pieces into the trash can.
7) As the pieces are thrown away, the practitioner helps the child connect with releasing the anxiety, worry, and dysregulated feelings.
8) This intervention can be repeated in future sessions, any time the child needs to take a feelings field trip.

Rationale

Feelings Field Trip helps children and adolescents work on increasing regulation, specifically decreasing anxious and worried feelings. This intervention can also be done focusing on angry feelings or other distressing thoughts. The practitioner processes through with the child that they can re-create this intervention any time at home or school when feeling worried or anxious. Parents are taught to do this intervention at home and encouraged to periodically complete the intervention with their child.

Music and Movement Feelings

Therapy Needs: Regulation, feeling identification and expression
Level: Child, adolescent
Materials: Several musical instruments
Modality: Individual

Introduction

Many neurodivergent children respond positively to music and movement. This play intervention incorporates music and movement with feeling identification and expression to help children improve regulation ability. The practitioner will need to have several different types of music producing instruments available for this intervention.

Instructions

1) The practitioner and child choose five feelings they are going to use in a music and dance performance they will create.
2) Once the feelings have been chosen, the child picks a musical instrument to go with each feeling.

3) The practitioner and child then decide on a dance or movement to go along with each feeling and instrument.
4) The child then decides the order of the performance.
5) The performance is then ready to begin. The practitioner and child play the instrument and perform the movement/dance for each feeling in the order the child has chosen. For example, the child chooses 'angry' to be the first feeling and chooses drums to be the instrument to represent the feeling, and chooses spinning around to be the dance/movement to represent angry. The practitioner and child both play the drums and spin around for a few seconds then move on to the second feeling/instrument/movement, and so forth until all five feelings have been performed.

Rationale

This play intervention helps children work on increasing regulation ability and identifying and expressing feelings. The focus is on helping a child identify troubling feelings that they are experiencing and demonstrating other ways to express those feelings (music and dance) other than verbally. It also incorporates sensory elements that help a child feel more relaxed after expressing a feeling. Parents can be taught to do this intervention at home and encouraged to role-play through negative feelings daily with their child.

Heart Parts

Therapy Needs: Regulation, feelings identification, anxiety reduction
Level: Child, adolescent
Materials: Foam pieces, black Sharpie, various craft decorations
Modality: Individual, family

Introduction

Neurodivergent children commonly struggle with anxiety and worry. High levels of anxiety and worry most often lead to a dysregulated system and unwanted behavior problems. Multiple sources can create high levels of anxiety in neurodivergent children such as social stressors, unexpected changes, new people or environments, sensory issues, trauma triggers, and inability to regulate emotions. This play intervention focuses on helping children identify anxiety and worry, and practice ways to regulate.

Instructions

1) The child selects a foam piece and cuts the foam piece into four different parts (practitioners can also have foam pieces available already cut into a heart shape).

2) The four parts are labeled: worried, loved, mad, and calm.
3) The practitioner and child begin with the worried part of the heart. The practitioner and child write on the front side of the heart part all the things they can think of that make the child feel worried. On the back side, the child and practitioner write strategies to help alleviate and regulate the negative feeling.
4) The same process is completed for the mad part of the heart.
5) The child takes the other two parts home and, together with their parents, writes all the things they can think of that make the child feel loved and calm on the loved and calm parts of the heart.
6) The child brings the completed parts back to the next session and the practitioner and child glue the heart together and process through the four different feelings, discussing what creates the feelings and helpful regulating strategies when experiencing negative feelings. The practitioner and child may want to role-play and practice the identified regulating strategies.

Rationale

Heart parts intervention works on feeling identification and regulation. The focus is on helping children to identify the feelings they have, what causes those feelings, and regulating strategies to address negative feelings. It also helps the child understand they can have different feelings, both positive and negative. The four feelings identified can be different from the four listed in this intervention but should always include positive and negative. Parents are taught to go through the two parts that are taken home with their child and further process through identifying and labeling feelings with their child.

Angry Yes, Peace Yes

Therapy Needs: Regulation, feeling identification
Level: Child, adolescent
Materials: White paper, construction paper, markers, glue, scissors
Modality: Individual

Introduction

The Angry Yes, Peace Yes intervention helps children and adolescents identify situations that make them feel angry or upset, and find peace-producing strategies or interventions to use to help them regulate or calm when something is dysregulating them. Any dysregulation, negative emotion, or experience can be addressed besides anger, such as worry, anxiety, frustration, disappointment, or sadness. The practitioner should target the intervention to address specific feelings and regulation needs the child is struggling with.

Instructions

1) The child is instructed to draw an outline of two people on a piece of white paper.
2) One person is labeled angry person and the other person is labeled peace person.
3) The practitioner informs the child that the people outlines represent the child.
4) The child picks a colored piece of construction paper for each person outline (one color for the angry person and one color for the peace person).
5) The child cuts out pieces of the colored paper and glues them on each person.
6) The child is instructed to write on the cut-out pieces of paper for the angry person the things that make them feel angry, and then to write on the cut-out pieces of paper for the peace person the things that make them feel peace. The practitioner may need to help the child identify things that make them feel angry and at peace.
7) The child then practices the things that make them feel at peace. The practitioner and child should role-play scenarios using situations or things that the child has identified as making them angry and then practicing a peace strategy.

Rationale

Peace work is an important construct that is often overlooked in working with children. Peace can create a state of mind that brings hope, which can be a powerful opposition to dysregulation. This play intervention helps children and adolescents work on identifying feelings and developing strategies to address dysregulation. Children should be encouraged to try and apply the peace strategies the next time they are feeling angry or dysregulated. The child can take this intervention home and practice the peace strategies there. Parents can also be taught how to do this intervention and practice with their child.

Spon-Play-Ity

Therapy Needs: Regulation, frustration tolerance, feelings identification
Level: Child, adolescent
Materials: Various toys and games
Modality: Individual

Introduction

Autistic, ADHD, and other neurodivergent children may struggle with changes in schedule or sudden spontaneous happenings. When this happens, it can create a great deal of dysregulation. This play intervention engages children in a playful way to practice regulating and coping when they experience sudden changes to a plan or experience something happening spontaneously without any preparation.

Instructions

1) The practitioner explains to the child that they will be working on how to better handle changes to a plan or something happening without any warning.
2) The practitioner asks the child to identify several games that they like to play. The games can be traditional boardgames or any type of game. If the child cannot think of anything, then the practitioner should make some suggestions of games to play that the child is familiar with.
3) The practitioner and child pick one of the identified games to start playing.
4) After about five minutes, the practitioner says to the child that they are not going to play that game any longer and chooses one of the other identified games to play.
5) The practitioner and child play the second game for about five minutes and then the practitioner again stops the game and chooses a different game to play.
6) This continues throughout most of the session. The practitioner may have to stop at times to help the child remember that they can regulate through the unexpected changes.
7) Toward the end of the session, the practitioner talks with the child about the process and asks them how it felt to keep changing without warning.
8) The practitioner and child then discuss the concept of things changing from the original plan and the concept of things happening spontaneously, and how the child can work on feeling okay and regulating through the changes.

Rationale

This play intervention provides the opportunity to regulate and mange frustration tolerance with things happening that are not planned or that change unexpectedly. The play therapy atmosphere proves a safe and regulating space to increase frustration tolerance. The practitioner and child may want to spend some time discussing ways to stay calm and regulate when things change, and try practicing those strategies during or before the intervention. The playful component of this intervention provides the child the opportunity to practice regulating themselves through changes in a less anxiety-stimulating context. Repetitive practice is important to help children become more comfortable with spontaneous events. The practitioner may want to implement this intervention across multiple sessions and teach parents how to implement this intervention at home.

Anxiety-Buster Toolbox

Therapy Needs: Regulation, anxiety reduction
Level: Child, adolescent
Materials: Small box, art supplies
Modality: Individual, group

Introduction

This play intervention provides a comprehensive tool for a child or adolescent to have available when they are feeling anxiety or dysregulated. It is likely that neurodivergent children will need many 'tools' to choose from to help them regulate. The anxiety-buster toolbox puts all the child's tools together in one accessible location where the child can choose what they need when they need it.

Instructions

1) The practitioner explains to the child that they will be making a box and placing in the box several ideas for helping the child calm and regulate when they are feeling anxious, upset, or overwhelmed.
2) The practitioner provides a small cardboard box for the child to decorate any way they would like. The child should write their name somewhere on the box.
3) Once the child has finished decorating the box, the practitioner instructs the child to cut several strips of paper. On each piece of paper, the practitioner and child will write things the child can do to help them regulate when they are feeling anxiety or dysregulated.
4) The practitioner will gain feedback from the child on what they believe helps them regulate. But, before this intervention is introduced, the practitioner should gain feedback from the child's parents, teachers, or any other people in the child's life who may be able to identify techniques, strategies, or games that currently help the child regulate when they are upset. The practitioner may also have some ideas for what might help the child and they can add those ideas to the box as well.
5) Once the box is complete, the practitioner and child should practice and role-play the regulation strategies. This may take multiple sessions. Also, new ideas and strategies can be added to the box at any time.
6) The child should take the box home and use as needed.

Rationale

This play intervention helps children and adolescents work on decreasing anxiety, regulating, and learning strategies to help them address a dysregulated system. Anything goes in the anxiety-buster toolbox that could be helpful to the child. Any activity, game, process, etc. that helps or may help a child calm or regulate can be written on a piece of paper and placed in the box. The box goes home with the child and the child is encouraged to go to their box and find something to do to help them regulate any time they are feeling dysregulated.

The Always-Changing Picture

Therapy Needs: Regulation, frustration tolerance, feelings identification
Level: Child, adolescent
Materials: Paper, markers, pencil
Modality: Individual, group, family

Introduction

Autistic and other neurodivergent children often need help in accepting transitions and managing when schedules and plans change. This intervention helps children practice handling changes and decreasing frustration tolerance in a low stimulating environment. It also helps teach children how to regulate though a distressing experience.

Instructions

1) The practitioner explains to the child that they are going to be working on helping the child handle experiencing change.
2) The practitioner explains that the child is going to draw a picture but there will be changes made to the picture as the child is drawing it.
3) The practitioner will begin by instructing the child to draw something; after a short time, the practitioner will change the instruction, giving a new instruction.
4) The practitioner will continue to do this several times before the final drawing is complete. An example might be, the practitioner tells the child to draw a house and color the roof blue. Halfway through the child coloring the roof blue, the practitioner changes the instruction to coloring the roof yellow. The practitioner might then instruct the child to draw a tree with leaves; as the child is drawing the leaves, the practitioner changes the instruction to no leaves. The practitioner will periodically give a new instruction, changing what was previously instructed.
5) This provides the child with the opportunity to practice accepting changes without becoming dysregulated. The practitioner can be processing with and talking to the child about how they are feeling as changes are being presented.
6) Once the drawing is complete, the practitioner and child can discuss what the process was like for the child.

Rationale

This play intervention helps children and adolescents practice regulating through situations and plans that change. The goal is to help children learn to 'switch gears' and stay calm and regulated through the changing process. By practicing in a lower stimulating 'safe' environment, such as a playroom with a play practitioner, the child can better prepare for real-life situations.

The practitioner should provide several changes to the original instruction, so the child has several opportunities to practice regulating through change in an atmosphere that is less dysregulating. The practitioner should process with the child staying calm and regulating through changes and applying examples to the child's real life.

Sand Games

Therapy Needs: Regulation, sensory needs, relationship development
Level: Child, adolescent
Materials: Sand tray, sand, various sand toys
Modality: Individual

Introduction

Sensory-different and other neurodivergent children may find sensory experiences regulating. Sand Games is a sensory-based intervention that helps children regulate and develop relationship connection. Some type of tub (sand tray) with soft sand should be used. Affirming note: Some children may have sensory sensitivity to sand. Alternatives can be used such as beans, rice, grass seed, or confetti.

Instructions

1) The practitioner explains to the child that they are going to be doing some activities in a sand tray.
2) The practitioner and child proceed in playing several sand games together.
   The practitioner and child take turns burying each other's hands and arms in the sand.
   The practitioner and child create a hand sand sifter, pouring sand from the practitioner's hand to the child's hand, back to the practitioner's hand.
   Hand cups: one person makes a hand cup and the other person fills it with sand.
   The practitioner and child each bury one hand in the sand and move their hand under the sand, trying to grab the other person's hand.
   The practitioner and child hold hands and place their held hands on top of the sand. With their free hands, the practitioner and child work together to bury the held hands in the sand.

3) The sand games can continue until the practitioner and child no longer want to play.

Rationale

The Sand Games intervention helps children work on regulation, connection, and relationship development. Children can discover a sensory-regulating experience and work on becoming more comfortable with interacting with another person and working with them to complete a task. This intervention can be repeated several times and the practitioner or child can create new sand games to play. Sand games should actively involve both the child and practitioner doing something together and/or utilizing the other person's hands/arms, etc. This intervention can be taught to parents to do at home with their child if the family can create a sand tray

Body Bubble Target

Therapy Needs: Regulation, social navigation, relationship development
Level: Child, adolescent
Materials: Bubbles
Modality: Individual, family, group

Introduction

Bubbles can provide a fun and sensory-pleasing process for many neurodivergent children. This play intervention uses bubbles in a game that promotes regulation, social navigation and connection, and relationship development. The practitioner will want to verify that the child does not mind getting touched by bubbles.

Instructions

1) The practitioner explains to the child that they will be playing a game that involves bubble blowing.
2) The practitioner and child decide who will blow the bubbles first. The other person will stand somewhere in the room and make a circle target with their arms and hands or any body part combination.
3) The bubble blower must stand a certain distance from the target (the practitioner can decide the appropriate distance). The bubble blower tries to blow as many bubbles as they can through the bubble target that the other person is making with their body parts.
4) After they have successfully blown several bubbles through the target, the practitioner and child can switch roles.
5) The practitioner and child can keep switching roles and playing the intervention throughout the whole session. Whoever is the target can change

the target position to vary the game. Some examples might include using your hands, arms, and legs to create a circle in front of the person, making a circle above the head, making a circle beside the body, making the circle larger or smaller, etc.

Rationale

This play intervention utilizes a bubble-blowing game to help children work on regulation, connection, and relationship development. This intervention also works on spatial and body awareness, and completing a game with another person. Parents can be taught how to implement this intervention at home and encouraged to play with their child and involve other family members.

Progressive Balloon Game

Therapy Needs: Regulation, social navigation, relationship development
Level: Child, adolescent
Materials: Balloon
Modality: Individual, family, group

Introduction

This play intervention utilizes a balloon game designed in video game fashion. The practitioner and child must progress through four levels of balloon hitting. This intervention is designed to be fun and interactive for the child and help address regulation needs. The practitioner will want to check with the child to make sure they do not have a balloon allergy and are not fearful of balloons before beginning this intervention.

Instructions

1) A balloon is blown up and tied off.
2) The practitioner explains that they are going to work together to progress through four levels and beat the balloon game.
3) The practitioner explains that each level will become a little more challenging, and through all four levels, they will work as a team to keep the balloon from hitting the ground.
4) The practitioner and child begin with Level One – hit the balloon back and forth any way you like. After a short amount of time, the practitioner announces they have progressed to Level Two.
5) The practitioner and child begin playing Level Two – put one arm/hand behind your back so you cannot use it. After a short amount of time, the practitioner announces they have progressed to Level Three.

6) The practitioner and child begin playing Level Three – put both arms/hands behind your back, you cannot use them. After a short amount of time, the practitioner announces they have progressed to Level Four.

7) The practitioner and child begin playing Level Four – you can only use your head, try to get ten hits. After ten hits, the practitioner announces they have beaten the game!

8) Throughout the game, if the balloon hits the ground, the practitioner should pick it up and put it back in play. The objective is to keep playing the game.

Rationale

This play intervention is designed to help children regulate their system, engage in a playful game with another person, and work with another person to complete a task. The game play should stay positive and fun. This intervention can also be done with families and groups.

10 Sensory Processing Interventions

Punching Bag Freestyle

Therapy Needs: Sensory needs, regulation
Level: Child, adolescent
Materials: Punching bag
Modality: Individual

Introduction

When children and adolescents are experiencing a great deal of dysregulation especially attached to frustration, anger, or anxiety, they can often benefit from a physical release to help them release and regulate. Punching Bag Freestyle provides a physical release and encourages children to discover experiences that are regulating for them.

Instructions

1) Using a punching bag, the practitioner explains to the child that they can explore the punching bag in any way they like.
2) The practitioner encourages the child to touch, hug, squeeze, punch, kick, sit on, lay on, etc. and discover what feels good for them.
3) The practitioner explains that many things can be done with a punching bag and the child is free to discover how to interact with a punching bag in ways that feel regulating for their system.
4) The practitioner allows the child to explore as long as they want.
5) As the child discovers different things that feel good to them, the practitioner can reinforce this as something the child can do when their system needs to explore regulation.

DOI: 10.4324/9781003398691-10

Rationale

This play intervention is designed to get children and adolescents exploring the possibilities of using a punching bag to provide a physical release for dysregulating states and emotions. The practitioner will want to make sure that the punching bag is age appropriate, safe, and durable (as some children and adolescents will hit the bag very hard). The practitioner may also want to provide a set of punching bag gloves for the child.

Noodle Relaxation Necklace

Therapy Needs: Sensory needs, regulation, anxiety reduction
Level: Child, adolescent
Materials: Swimming pool noodle, string, scissors
Modality: Individual, group

Introduction

The Noodle Relaxation Necklace intervention functions as an assistive device for children to help them regulate in a way that can be more socially acceptable. Neurodivergent children can often benefit from finding an appropriate device or action to manipulate to help them regulate and stay calm when they are feeling dysregulated or anxious. This play intervention provides the creation of a fun necklace to serve as a regulating item.

Instructions

1) Using a swimming pool noodle, the practitioner and child cut three small pieces off the noodle.
2) The child chooses three different colors and then puts the pieces on a piece of string that is then tied around the child's neck. Figure 10.1 provides a noodle relaxation necklace example.
3) The necklace should be loose enough so the child can put it on and take it off easily.
4) The practitioner explains to the child that they can squeeze and grab the noodle pieces as much and as hard as they want, any time they feel anxious, stressed, or upset in any way.
5) The practitioner and child decide on a relaxation reminder that will go with each color. Some examples include: 'It will be okay,' 'I have friends,' and 'I can do this.'

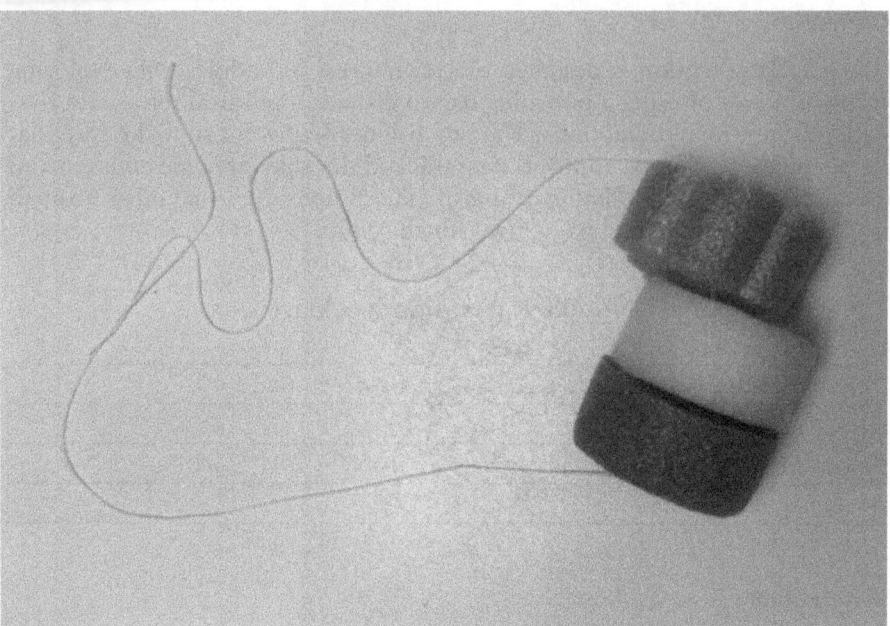

Figure 10.1 Pool noodle necklace example.

Robert Jason Grant

6) The practitioner and child can practice using the necklace and the child gets to take the necklace home and the child can wear the necklace or keep it in their room or backpack.
7) This intervention also makes for a great classroom project. The whole class can learn to make the necklaces and anyone can wear them any time they want.

Rationale

This play intervention provides a fun and helpful tool for regulation. Multiple necklaces can be made to be kept in various locations and if something happens to a necklace, a new one can be easily made. Practitioners should caution that the noodle pieces cannot be bitten or chewed on.

Clay Away

Therapy Needs: Sensory needs, regulation, relaxation
Level: Child, adolescent
Materials: Clay or playdough
Modality: Individual, group

Introduction

The Clay Away intervention uses clay or a related material to provide a sensory experience that helps children and adolescents relax and work through worries and anxiety. Several anxiety-producing situations can be processed through with this intervention.

Instructions

1) The child is instructed to think about a time or situation when they have felt anxious or worried.
2) Using modeling clay, the child is instructed to think about the time or situation that made them feel anxious and press their fingers into the clay. After a couple of minutes, the child is instructed to press their palms into the clay. After a couple of minutes, their fists into the clay.
3) The child is then instructed to grab the clay in their hands and try to squish it.
4) The child is then instructed to put the clay on the table and try to smash it with their fists (a small rubber mallet can also be used).
5) Finally, the child is instructed to make something out of the clay that reminds them of or makes them feel happy or calm.

Rationale

Clay Away provides children and adolescents with a sensory-based experience to recognize and process through times and situations that produce anxiety and worry for them. The practitioner should have the child manipulate the clay for about ten minutes before they create something that makes them feel happy or calm. The practitioner should process through with the child after have completed the intervention on how it felt to think about their anxiety while manipulating the clay and how it felt to create something that represented a happy or calm feeling.

Build Around Me

Therapy Needs: Sensory needs, regulation, body awareness, connection	
Level: Child, adolescent	
Materials: Cardboard bricks or large foam blocks	
Modality: Individual, family	

Introduction

Autistic, sensory-different, and other neurodivergent children can often feel comforted by weight pressing upon them. This play intervention provides a playful way to give children a weighted and released sensory experience and provides a fun connection element.

Instructions

1) The child will sit or lay down on the floor.
2) The practitioner will take cardboard bricks or large foam blocks and build something around and over the child. The child will be mostly or completely covered in bricks or blocks.
3) The child is instructed to try and sit or lay still under the bricks for a few seconds.
4) Once the practitioner has finished, the child is given a countdown and instructed to bust out!
5) The intervention can be repeated as long as the child wants to play.

Rationale

This play intervention helps children and adolescents work on sensory, regulation, connection, and impulse control/body awareness. The practitioner should present the intervention to the child and make sure the child wants to participate and understands that they will be covered in bricks or blocks. The intervention can be repeated many times. The practitioner should try to engage the child to switch roles and have the child build something around the practitioner. The intervention can be taught to parents to do at home with their child. Cardboard bricks and large foam blocks can be found at most major toy stores or online toy sites.

Regulation Ball

Therapy Needs: Sensory needs, regulation, relaxation
Level: Child, adolescent
Materials: Beach ball, marker
Modality: Individual, group, family

Introduction

Relaxation Ball provides a playful and engaging game for children to identify and practice coping skills and relaxation techniques to use when they are feeling anxious or dysregulated. A blown-up beach ball is used and can be individualized to a child's needs.

Instructions

1) Before the session, the practitioner takes a blown-up beach ball and, with a black marker, writes things on the beach ball that the child can do to help them calm down, relax, or regulate. Table 10.1 provides some examples for regulating activities to write on the ball.

Table 10.1 Regulation Ball Examples

Take five deep breaths
Play patty cake
Do some exercises
Punch a punching bag
Talk about your favorite game to play
Walk in slow motion across the room
Tell and joke and laugh
Count backwards from 100 by 7
Hop on one foot around the room
Walk backwards around the room
Say your name backwards

Source: Grant, R. J. (2023).

2) During the session, the practitioner and child pass the beach ball back and forth and, when the ball is caught, whatever is written closest to the person's right thumb is what the person reads and will complete.
3) Play continues until all the things on ball have been practiced or until the practitioner and child no longer want to play.
4) After the session, the practitioner can give the ball to the child to take home and play with their parents.
5) When deciding upon what to write on the ball, the practitioner should first consult with the child's parents about what things typically help the child regulate, calm, or relax. The practitioner can also explore this with the child and add new ideas to the ball.

Rationale

This play intervention is designed to help children and adolescents work on learning strategies to help regulate, calm, and relax. Ideally, the regulation ball is sent home with the child for the parents and child to play this intervention at home together. Parents and children can play several times a week. This can even become a part of the child's regulation lifestyle, ensuring they have regulating experiences in their day and week.

I Sense Story

Therapy Needs: Sensory needs, regulation
Level: Child, adolescent
Materials: Paper, pencil, various toys
Modality: Individual, family, group

Introduction

I Sense Story works on helping children to identify and practice working on sensory processing needs in a way that is playful and promotes relationship development, coping skills, and regulation. This activity is designed to engage multiple sensory areas and can be repeated multiple times with a new story each time.

Instructions

1) The practitioner gives the instructions to the child that the child will be writing a poem and creating a visual activity to go with the poem.
2) The poem is a sentence completion based on the eight sensory areas. It is written as follows: Looks like... Sounds like... Smells like... Tastes like... Feels like... Moves like...
3) The child completes each sentence based on a visual or activity in the playroom. An example would be: Sounds like a musical instrument. The child would identify a musical instrument in the playroom and complete the line, based on identifying the musical instrument.
4) Once the child is finished, the child reads the poem and performs the activity that goes with each line of the poem. In the example, the child would read, 'Sounds like a musical instrument,' and the child would play the selected musical instrument while reading the line.
5) The practitioner allows the child to write the whole poem and select an activity for each line of the poem (each sensory area) and offers help only if the child indicates they need help. The practitioner can join the child and they can complete the poem/activity together.

Rationale

This play intervention is helpful for children and adolescents who are experiencing dysregulation or anxiety due to sensory needs. When creating the story, the practitioner should be sensitive to specific sensory challenges the child struggles with and may suggest activities to go with each line of the poem that might be helpful for the child to practice or work on, such as, 'Feels like a back brush,' for children who find it calming to be brushed. An I Sense Story worksheet is provided in the Appendix.

I Sense Story Example

Looks like funny glasses (child finds some funny glasses and puts them on while reading this line).

Sounds like a musical instrument (child finds a musical instrument and plays it while reading this line).

Smells like a dry erase marker (child gets a dry erase marker and smells it while reading this line).

Tastes like a piece of candy (child gets a piece of candy and tastes it while reading this line). Feels like sand in the sand tray (child puts hands in the sand tray while reading this line).

Moves like a monkey (child moves around the room like a monkey while reading this line).

Balancing Act

(Contributed by Cary M. Hamilton, Registered Play Therapist Supervisor™)

Therapy Needs: Sensory needs, regulation
Level: Child
Materials: Bop bag, floor space
Modality: Individual

Introduction

This play intervention involves using a bop bag. These types of bags are commonplace in most play therapy rooms, as they provide a safe way for a child to release their anger, aggression, and energy. Bop bags are weighted at the bottom, which allows them to pop back upright after a child knocks them over. Bop bags can be used in many ways and this activity highlights one way to structure a bop bag activity to improve sensory processing needs.

Instructions

1) The practitioner explains to the child that they will be doing an activity to strengthen their muscles and release tension in their bodies.
2) The practitioner explains that they will be using a bop bag and clears a large space in the room (large enough for the bop bag to tip over).
3) The practitioner encourages the child to hit, punch, or kick the bop bag X number of times (the number of times can reflect the child's age or be increased/decreased based on the child's need for sensory input). The child can continue to hit, punch, or kick the bop bag until they are no longer interested.
4) The practitioner then encourages the child to run at the bop bag to knock it down. Once the bop bag is on the floor, the child is encouraged to get on the bop bag and find their balance on the bag, so they do not roll off onto the floor. The child can repeat the running, knocking down, and finding their balance portion of this activity any number of times until balance is achieved. Figure 10.2 provides an example.

Rationale

Sensory-different and other neurodivergent children can often struggle with core stability, which would help their bodies with gross motor skills, fine motor skills, balance, and coordination of movement. Balancing tasks are a great way to help a child work on building their core stability while achieving a goal. A bop bag is typically used to release challenging emotions and aggression; using a bop bag in this way also works on a child's proprioceptive sense, which

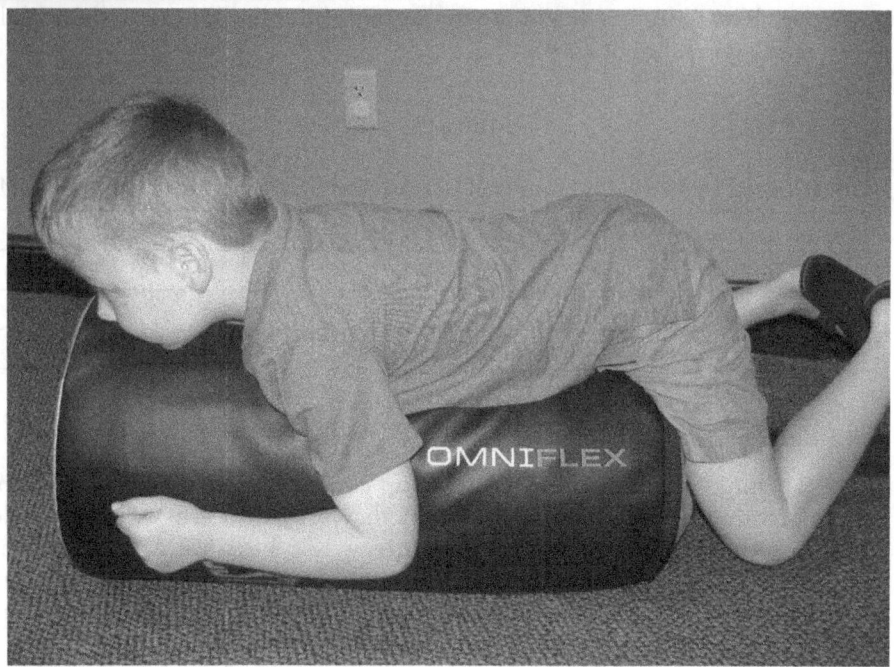

Figure 10.2 Balancing act example.
Robert Jason Grant

focuses on the movement of muscles and joints. Adding on the balance component is an easy way to incorporate both sensory target areas. Practitioners may
find this activity beneficial to use with children who arrive at a session dysregulated, or are frequently seeking sensory input from climbing, jumping, and
moving. Parents can easily purchase a bop bag to have at home for the child to
use whenever they need regulation work, or parents can structure time with the
bop bag such as implementing this balancing act intervention.

Burrito Roll

(Contributed by Cary Hamilton, Registered Play Therapist Supervisor™)

Therapy Needs: Sensory needs, regulation
Level: Child, adolescent
Materials: Weighted blanket
Modality: Individual, family

Introduction

A weighted blanket is used to complete this activity. Weighted blankets are
regular blankets that have been weighted to feel heavier when used by a

person. These blankets provide pressure and sensory input for individuals with sensory differences. A weighted blanket can be used as a calming tool as the pressure of the blanket provides proprioceptive input to the brain. This activity is helpful for sensory work and emotion regulation. Practitioners might find this activity helpful before and/or after a session where abreaction is present.

Instructions

1) The practitioner explains to the child that they will be doing an activity to help regulate their body and they will be using a weighted blanket (the practitioner should show the child the weighted blanket and let them feel it before beginning the activity).
2) The practitioner lays a weighted blanket down on the floor and asks the child to lay down on top of it.
3) The practitioner then wraps the child up in the weighted blanket and instructs the child to lay still for several minutes; the practitioner may lay down next to the child to cause less distraction and/or get on the child's physical level if it helps the child feel more comfortable.
4) The practitioner then asks the child if they would like to be rolled across the floor in the weighted blanket; some children may be more open to this than others. If the child would like to be rolled across the floor, the practitioner will do this a few times until the child is no longer interested. Figure 10.3 provides an example.

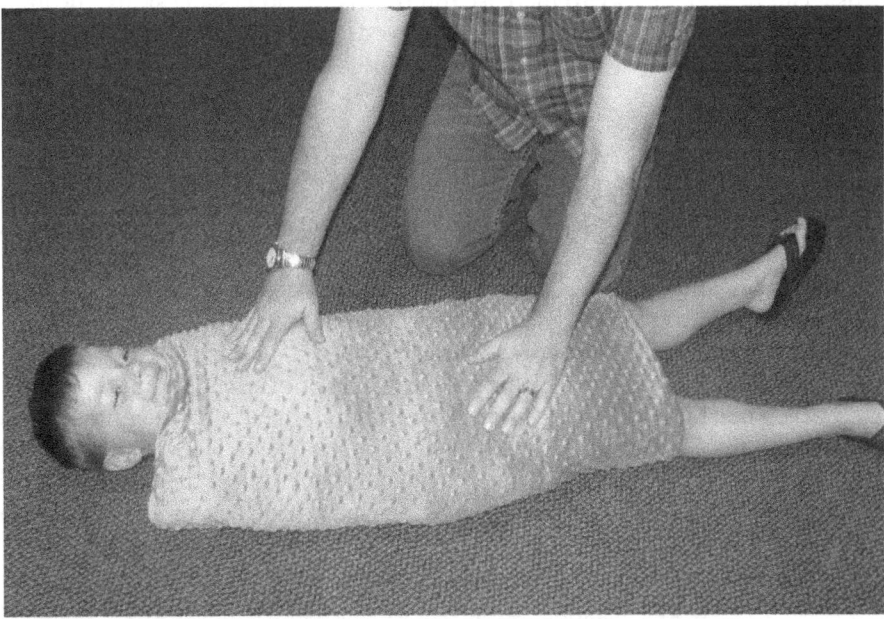

Figure 10.3 Burrito roll example.

Robert Jason Grant

Rationale

Weighted blankets work to help children regulate their bodies, and in turn calm their minds. The pressure of weighted blankets is beneficial to children who seek greater amounts of tactile input (hyporesponsive). This activity allows for body regulation, particularly for children coming to therapy after school and those with ADHD symptoms. Having the parent assist allows for it to become a connecting exercise and ease transitions. Parents can implement this activity regularly at home to help their child stay regulated.

Bring On the Music

(Contributed by Amy Vaughan OTR/L, BCP from *Positively Sensory: A Guide to Help your Child Develop Positive Approaches to Learning and Cope with Sensory Processing Difficulty*)

Therapy Needs: Sensory needs, regulation, executive functioning needs
Level: Child, adolescent
Modality: Individual, family
Materials Needed: Dry erase board, dry erase markers, music player, relaxing music.

Introduction

Music can be a great way to increase multi-sensory processing skills, the ability to filter information, and the ability to attend and shift attention. This activity aims to create a see it/hear it/do it loop for learning.

Instructions

1) The practitioner explains to the child or adolescent they will be doing an activity that involves drawing on a dry erase board and listening to music.
2) The practitioner draws a shape on a dry erase board and has the child look at it and name it. The practitioner then covers the shape, and the child must draw it from memory. This is done until the child can successfully remember and draw five shapes.
3) The practitioner uses their finger to draw one of the shapes on the child's back. The child will picture it in their mind, name it, and then draw it on the dry erase board.
4) The practitioner will add music (typically something relaxing such as Beethoven or the child's choice) and repeat the above sequence while the music is playing.
5) With the music continuing to play, the practitioner will use their finger to draw two shapes in relationship to one another on the child's back. The child will picture it in their mind and then draw it on the dry erase board.

6) The practitioner will switch from shapes to letters and keep repeating the activity until the activity time is over.

Rationale

Music can be a powerful tool. It can bypass our natural avenues for taking in information through regular pathways in the brain and often enters through our emotions. Using music for therapeutic change can be very powerful. Music can support and enhance the child's ability to engage in daily routines. Providing auditory cues in preparation for a transition can be as helpful as visual scheduling. This activity uses music to help children with sensory needs and executive functioning issues. The activity can be played regularly to strengthen both sensory and executing functioning needs.

Fun With Your Feet

(Contributed by Kim Vander Dussen Registered Play Therapist Supervisor™)

Therapy Needs: Sensory needs
Level: Child, adolescent
Materials: An assortment of surfaces of 10–12 different textures that can be walked on, some are more pleasing than others to allow for a diversity of sensory experiences. For example, be sure to include a soft fleece blanket, a grass doormat, bubble wrap, a pillow cover filled with beans, a pillow cover filled with packing peanuts, a bamboo place mat, a coarse wool blanket, etc. These items should be arranged in a circle with sufficient distance so that you can only occupy one surface at a time. Music will also be played.
Modality: Individual, family, group

Introduction

Children with sensory differences often struggle with distal body parts like hands and feet. It is also common for the processing difficulties to be multi-sensory in nature. In order to help children with these processing needs, it is important to engage them in fun, pleasurable activities that have been shown to help decrease anxiety associated with hypersensitivities.

Instructions

1) The practitioner explains to the child or adolescent they will be doing an activity that involves a twist on the traditional game of musical chairs. Instead of moving from chair to chair, they will be walking across different surfaces barefoot or with socks only (dependent upon the intensity of sensitivity). Instructions should include something like 'Some of these

surfaces will feel really good and may even be fun, and some will feel a little bit uncomfortable.'

2) The practitioner may or may not participate in the play. This should be the child's choice. Allowing the child or teen to control some decision making is an empowering process.

3) The practitioner then explains that when the music is playing, the child will be moving steadily across the different surfaces. Encourage the child to identify when they do or don't like a texture. When the music stops, the child must stand still on a surface, while one of the unused ones is removed. Figure 10.4 provides an example.

4) The practitioner should choose music with at least 80 beats per minute. Music with a distinctly positive message like 'Happy' by Pharrell, 'Can't Stop the Feeling' by Justin Timberlake, 'Love Shack' by the B-52s, or 'Walk This Way' by Run DMC are regulating and improve mood.

5) With the music continuing to play, the practitioner will stop and start the song as if they are playing musical chairs, with the surfaces becoming increasingly limited (for group or family work, individuals are being eliminated from the game when spaces run out until a winner remains on the sole surface left).

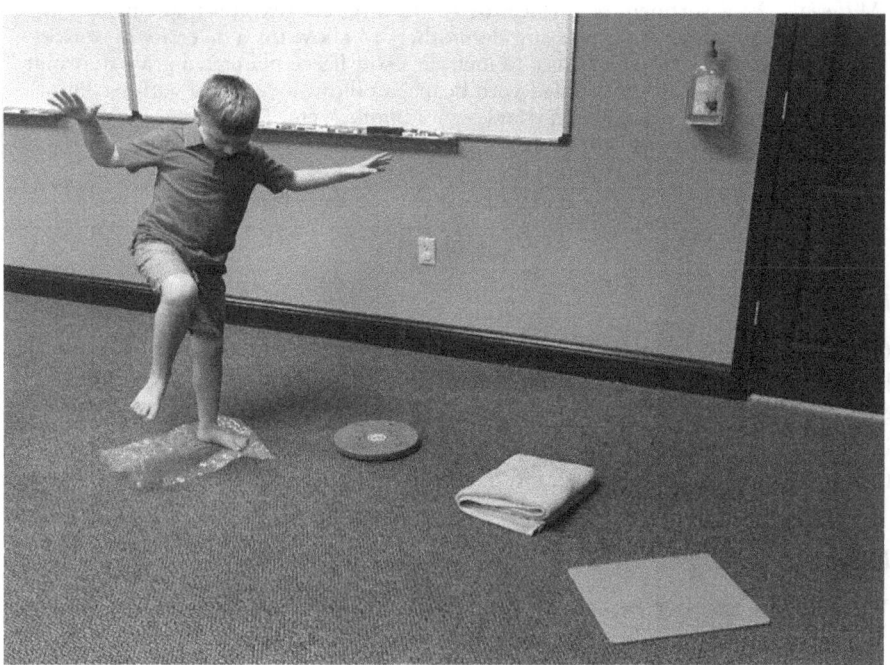

Figure 10.4 Fun with your feet example.

Robert Jason Grant

Rationale

Sensory processing differences reflect fundamental brain functioning. Activities like Fun With Your Feet are designed to promote healthier brain functioning. The most adaptive interventions are relational (which makes people feel safe), rhythmic (which is consistent with brain patterns), repetitive (follows a predictable pattern), relevant (consistent with developmental level), rewarding (fun!), and respectful (mindful of culture, the family, and the child).

Digging Deeper

(Contributed by Mistie Barnes Registered Play Therapist™)

Therapy Needs: Sensory needs, regulation, relationship development
Level: Child
Materials: Sand tray (or other container), sand (hypoallergenic is best)
Modality: Individual, family, group

Introduction

The goal of this play intervention is to allow the opportunity to engage in and build tolerance to three forms of tactile stimulation (temperature, touch, and sand stimulation), while engaging in rapport and relationship building. Parents can be involved by encouraging them to be actively engaged in the 'digging' process. This process allows the parent to build rapport with their child on two levels; by interacting with their child in the digging process, as well as through the medium of touch as they work to uncover the child's fingers in the sand. The act of gently brushing the sand from the skin can be a bonding experience between child and adult.

Instructions

1) The practitioner begins by introducing the child to the sand tray and sand.
2) The practitioner encourages the child to become familiar and comfortable with the sand through touch, sound (listening as the sand runs through their fingers), and visually.
3) When comfortable, the child is encouraged to bury their hands as deep as they feel comfortable in the sand, and as much of their hands and fingers as they feel comfortable burying. (Note: Some may bury their fingers, their hands, and even part of their arms.)
4) The practitioner encourages the child to experience the temperature of the sand; the coolness (or warmth if heated) of the sand against their fingers, against the top and bottom of their hand, and as it touches their wrists.

5) The practitioner suggests the child move their hand(s) and finger(s) in the sand, wiggle them around, and feel the sand moving on and around their hands and fingers, feeling the sand move around, and experiencing the texture of individual pieces of sand.

6) After the child has had time to experience the temperature and feel of the sand, they are again encouraged to re-bury their hands and fingers in the sand as deep as they feel comfortable.

7) After the child has buried their hands and fingers and feels comfortable, the practitioner will begin working in the sand. The practitioner will gently move the sand aside slowly, as they work to uncover the child's hand. As the practitioner digs down in the sand, they will brush aside the sand as it covers the child's hand and fingers, allowing the child to experience the feeling of fresh air now touching their skin, and the gentle touch of the adult gently removing the sand from their hands and fingers.

8) The child will tell the practitioner when their hands and fingers are completely found, and they are ready to start over – for some, they may choose to be free at the first sign of skin; for others, they may choose to wait until the practitioner has completely uncovered their entire hand and all fingers.

9) The practitioner may choose to ask some processing questions such as, 'What does the sand feel like?' 'Is it a good feeling or a not good feeling?' 'How deep do you want your fingers and hands to go?' 'Does it feel better for your hands to be closer to the top, or closer to the bottom?' 'What makes it feel better for your hands to be closer to the top/bottom?' 'What does it feel like to move through the sand?' 'When waiting for the practitioner to unbury your hands and fingers, what did this feel like?' 'Tell me about the feelings you felt in your fingers when the practitioner was uncovering them?' 'Tell me about the feelings you felt in your hands when the practitioner was uncovering them?' 'What were the feelings you felt in your body while the practitioner was uncovering your hands and fingers?'

Rationale

This play intervention is designed to build rapport between the practitioner and child. It also builds relationship between the parent and child. This intervention allows the opportunity to engage in three types of tactile stimulation and increases tolerance to three types of tactile stimulation. This activity is designed to be used with individuals (with the practitioner as the one digging for the hands and fingers) and family (with the parent digging for the hands and fingers).

This play intervention can be adapted to a group setting by presenting additional sand trays and allowing group members to work with one another. One individual will bury their hands and fingers, while the second individual works to dig their hands and fingers out of the sand. This intervention can be adapted to a family group setting by providing additional sand trays and assigning each family group to their own sand tray. The family groups will then complete the intervention based on the general directions. Children may choose to cover not only their fingers and hands, but they may also choose to cover part of their arms. Some children may be uncomfortable with the texture of the sand. Other options might be rice, beans, or a quantity of other small objects. Affirming note: Some children will have sensory differences related to sand or other substances. Also, when working in high poverty areas, working with food items may not be appropriate, as individuals who are dealing with poverty issues may experience discomfort working and playing with food items.

What Do I Like and Not Like?

(Contributed by Natascha Lawrence BC Registered Play Therapist)

Therapy Needs: Sensory needs, regulation, and connection.
Level: Child, adolescent
Materials: Selection of sensory materials that engage each of the sensory systems, such as:

1. Visual (sight) – bright lights, LED lights, soft lighting
2. Gustatory (taste) – mints, lemon, hot chocolate, hot sauce
3. Tactile (touch) – rough rocks, soft fabric
4. Auditory (hearing) – selection of instruments, songs from different genres of music
5. Olfactory (smell) – lavender, lemons, vanilla
6. Vestibular (balance) – balance board, spinning chair
7. Proprioceptive (movement) – heavy bean bags, light feathers
8. Interoceptive (internal) – warm drink, ice

Modality: Individual, family, group

Introduction

Neurodivergent children and adolescents may have difficulty interpreting and organizing input from their sensory systems. This play intervention can be easily adapted for individual needs. It is a fun, exploratory activity requiring a variety of materials, but these materials can be easily found within existing playrooms, in nature, or brought from home. They do not have to be expensive. This play intervention can encourage the practitioner to be creative and find new materials to explore the different sensory systems. To promote investigation and the exploration of various concepts during sensory play, the practitioner should aim to provide resources that offer contrasting experiences (i.e., heavy versus light, cold versus hot, dark versus bright).

Instructions

1) The practitioner explains to the child they are going to play a game where the child will get to explore their sensory preferences (what they like and what they do not like).

2) The practitioner can introduce the eight sensory systems: visual (sight), gustatory (taste), tactile (touch), auditory (hearing), olfactory (smell), vestibular (balance), proprioceptive (movement), interoceptive (internal)

3) The practitioner presents different materials to engage each sensory system. It is encouraged that one sensory system is focused on at a time, with two to three materials only, to avoid overstimulation. Different materials can be presented in separate sessions.

4) The practitioner can start with lighting preferences in the playroom, such as dimmed, bright, or lights off.

5) The practitioner allows the child to explore the materials independently. The practitioner provides gentle encouragement but ensures that the child can choose to engage with a material or not.

6) The practitioner tracks the sensory play, providing feedback on the child's engagement, somatic responses, verbalizations, and reactions. The practitioner and child can also write down or make a visual representation of the sensory preferences. The practitioner and child can decide how they would want to share this information with parents, teachers, and other supports. The practitioner and child can create a sensory toolkit with preferred materials for the playroom, home, or at school.

7) The practitioner can introduce the sensory system of interoception. The practitioner can ask the child how they know that they like or do not like each material. Other play interventions can be added to deepen the understanding of how the child knows how they feel.

8) The play continues as long as the child wants. The play can continue into subsequent sessions, and can include looking for other sensory exploration materials, in the playroom, at home, or in nature.

Rationale

Children learn more from interacting with their environment than from passive observation or learning. Sensory play encourages and facilitates the development and integration of the senses. Sensory exploration plays a vital role in interoceptive development, the perception of sensations inside the body. Interoception is crucial in understanding how we feel and if we need to use a strategy to regulate.

As neurodivergent children can often have difficulty interpreting and organizing sensory input, one or more sensory systems may be over- or under-reactive to stimulation. Overstimulation can cause distress, anxiety, overwhelm, and even pain. Under-stimulation can cause anxiety, irritation, difficulty concentrating, and dissociation.

It is beneficial for neurodivergent children to learn their sensory preferences to find the best way to use self-soothing and stimming to regulate. Neurodivergent children can benefit from having a tailored sensory diet based on their preferences and unique sensory needs. Understanding their sensory needs can allow children to communicate and advocate for these needs in different settings, such as in the playroom, at home, school, and in the community. A practitioner can use preferred sensory materials in other play interventions and to help deepen regulation in the playroom. The practitioner and child can create a sensory toolkit that can be replicated and easily accessible in areas where over- or under-stimulation can occur. A variation of this play intervention can be integrated at the beginning of sessions to ensure that the playroom and waiting room are set up to meet the child's sensory needs (i.e., lighting preferences, scent preferences, sound preferences).

Angry Elephant Stomps

(Contributed by Emma N. Arnoff Licensed Clinical Social Worker)

Therapy Needs: Sensory needs, regulation, feeling identification
Level: Child, adolescent
Materials: None
Modality: Individual, family, group

Introduction

Autistic and other neurodivergent children can benefit from sensory input and movement. This activity combines sensory integration, movement, and emotional regulation. This intervention supports children in identifying and expressing their anger with the goal of helping them regulate. This play intervention involves movement play and it requires no materials. It can be easily implemented in any setting.

Instructions

1) The practitioner explains to the child that they will be stomping like elephants.
2) The practitioner shows the child how they stomp like an elephant by lifting their foot high in the air and stomping hard on the floor.
3) The practitioner asks the child to try and encourages them to stomp as hard as they can.
4) The practitioner checks in on how this feels for the child.
5) The practitioner explains they will be stomping out what makes them angry. The practitioner shares an example of something that makes them angry (traffic, weather, etc.).

6) The practitioner shows the child how to put their angry thought on the floor and elephant stomp on it.
7) The practitioner asks the child to think of something that makes them angry. If the child is willing and able, they can share this.
8) The child puts their angry thought on the floor and stomps on it.
9) The child repeats this with further angry thoughts.
10) The intervention goes on until the child is no longer interested. Once the play is completed, the practitioner checks in with the child to see how this intervention felt for them.

Rationale

This play intervention supports Autistic and other neurodivergent children in regulating their bodies, identifying their emotions, and releasing their anger. This intervention is playful and engaging, which helps build the therapeutic relationship. This intervention can be used in groups or taught to parents to use at home.

Sick Ball Obstacle Course

(Contributed by Danyale Weems Registered Play Therapist Supervisor™)

Therapy Needs: Sensory needs, regulation
Level: Child
Materials: Cones, sock balls, swimming noodles (at least two full noodles cut in half), long tube socks rolled up like a hair bun
Modality: Individual, family

Introduction

Sensory-different and other neurodivergent children may have sensory and regulation needs. These children may experience sensory processing at a higher rate than the general population. These needs can impact the family system and their environments. This play intervention aims to help children who struggle with sensory areas through providing a fun, low-challenge physical movement to improve their awareness of their bodies in their environment.

Instructions

1) The practitioner sets up cones outside (or in a big room), using several to create an obstacle course.
2) The practitioner places pool noodles (cut in half) throughout the course.
3) The child is at one end of the course and the practitioner is at the other end.

4) The child runs through the course (not moving any cones or pool noodles) once, with no time limit.
5) The child runs the course a second time, being timed.
6) The child runs the course a third time with balls being tossed toward the child by the practitioner. The child dodges the balls while completing the course, leaving no cone turned and no pool noodle moved.
7) The practitioner can add elements to the course such as moving fast, slow, and stopping instructions.
8) The practitioner can provide coaching as needed throughout the course and provide the child with choices once they have experienced the various options. The practitioner and child can create a new course with new instructions for completing the course.
9) The intervention is played until the practitioner and child are no longer interested.

Rationale

This play intervention will assist with sensory needs, regulation, connection, and relationship development. It provides a fun, physical movement game format. It can be done in sessions with the practitioner and also with the child and their parents as a family intervention or as a group intervention.

11 Connection and Relationship Development Interventions

Obstacle Course

Therapy Needs: Connection, relationship development
Level: Child, adolescent
Materials: Several pieces of paper
Modality: Individual, family, group

Introduction

Autistic and other neurodivergent children may struggle with comfort in interacting with others. Anxiety, previous rejecting experiences, and trauma triggers may all be struggles when engaging with others. Natural and affirming play interventions can help children feel more regulated and gain enjoyment in connecting with others. This intervention helps children work on connection, trust, being present with another person, and general relationship development.

Instructions

1) The practitioner explains to the child that they will be playing a game to work on trusting and becoming more comfortable with other people.
2) The practitioner wads up several pieces of paper and places them around the playroom.
3) The practitioner then explains to the child that they are going to take turns leading each other from one side of the playroom to the other without stepping on any of the pieces of paper, and that the person being led will be wearing a blindfold.
4) The practitioner goes first and blindfolds the child. The practitioner stands behind the child with their hands on the child's shoulders. The practitioner should check in with the child first and make sure they are comfortable being blindfolded and are comfortable with the practitioner putting their hands on their shoulders. This intervention can also be done with having the child close their eyes and with no touch, just verbal prompts.

DOI: 10.4324/9781003398691-11

5) The practitioner guides the child with words and physical prompts across the playroom, having the child avoid stepping on any of the pieces of paper.
6) Once successfully across the playroom, the practitioner and child switch roles and the child leads the practitioner back across the playroom, avoiding all the pieces of paper.
7) The game can be played multiple times with the paper being re-arranged each time. The practitioner should regularly check in with the child to make sure they are feeling comfortable with the game.

Rationale

This play intervention helps children and adolescents work on connection and relationship development. Children and adolescents can work on becoming more comfortable with engaging other people and working on reducing any anxiety that might accompany interacting with others. The practitioner and child can play the intervention several times. Each time they play, they can mix up the pieces of paper on the floor so there is a new obstacle field to guide through. Parents can be taught this intervention to implement at home and be encouraged to play regularly with their child and include the entire family. This intervention, along with several of the connection interventions, requires a level of physical touch. This should always be explained to the child before implementation and the practitioner should confirm with the child that they feel comfortable with the level of touch and close proximity of the practitioner.

Lizard Walk

Therapy Needs: Connection, relationship development, attachment, sensory needs
Level: Child
Materials: None
Modality: Individual, family

Introduction

Lizard Walk is a simple yet effective intervention that helps children develop relationship and connection with others. It is presented in a fun and playful manner that engages children to participate. Further, it helps children understand and become comfortable with positive touch, closely interacting with another person, and can serve as a sensory-affirming intervention.

Instructions

1) The practitioner tells the child that the practitioner is going to do a lizard walk up and down the child's arms and legs.

2) The practitioner should demonstrate on a stuffed animal or the practitioner's own arm first to show the child what will be happening and gain the child's consent.

3) The child sits on the floor or a chair and holds out one arm. The practitioner makes their hands into the formation of talking puppet hands, and one hand at a time, the practitioner clamps onto the child's hand (starting with the child's fingers) and moves up the child's arms, clamping onto the child as a lizard might clamp on and walk up the child's arm.

4) The practitioner then repeats the same action for the child's other arm and then the child's legs.

5) The practitioner can then ask the child if they want to do the lizard walk on the practitioner. The practitioner should be cautious to explain to the child that there will be touch involved and gain permission from the child for each level of touch.

6) The practitioner and child can play Lizard Walk back and forth several times.

Rationale

This play intervention helps children work on connection and relationship development, especially in attuning to others, becoming comfortable with physical touch, and participating in a reciprocal activity with another person. This intervention also serves as a sensory-regulating and co-regulating intervention that can be done with the child. This intervention can be repeated several times. The practitioner should encourage the child to complete the lizard walk on the practitioner, but if the child is not comfortable with this, it should not be forced. This intervention works well as a family play intervention and can be taught to parents to do regularly at home with their child. This connection intervention can be paired with other connection interventions for parents to do with their child at home and involve the entire family.

Feeling Card Find It

Therapy Needs: Connection, relationship development, feeling identification
Level: Child, adolescent
Materials: Index cards, pencil
Modality: Individual, family

Introduction

Neurodivergent children may have needs with feeling safe and comfortable connecting with others. Connection often includes both social navigation and emotional components. This intervention helps children develop relationship connection, social navigation, and emotional regulation. The practitioner can design this intervention to address specific feelings that the child may need help in expressing and regulating.

Instructions

1) The practitioner and child write feeling words on several index cards (usually 8–10 to begin with).
2) The practitioner and child then take turns picking an index card and hiding it somewhere on their body while the other person is not watching.
3) The other person then has to find the card on the person's body by physically searching for it.
4) Once the card is found, the person who found it has to read the feeling word on the card and talk about something that makes them feel that way.
5) This process is repeated until all the index cards have been completed.
6) The practitioner should hide the cards in fairly obvious places on their body. If the child is uncomfortable with being touched or touching the practitioner, then words can be used and each person can point at different areas on the body.

Rationale

This play intervention helps children work on connection and relationship development, social navigation and feeling identification and awareness. This intervention can be repeated several times, with the practitioner and child creating different feeling index cards. Placement of index cards on the body should be somewhat obvious, such as coming out of a sleeve, on top of head, coming out of shoe, etc. This intervention helps children learn to notice and attune to another person, recognize and express feelings, and develop connection. The practitioner can also change the feeling share time to another instruction, such as define the feeling. This intervention works well as a family play intervention and can be taught to parents to do at home with their child. Parents are encouraged to attune to what their child may be feeling and represent those feelings in the index feeling cards. Parents are also encouraged to involve the entire family.

Ring Around Me

Therapy Needs: Connection, relationship development, attachment
Level: Child
Materials: None
Modality: Individual, family

Introduction

Ring Around Me is a fun and engaging connection intervention, especially for young children. Physical contact is maintained throughout the activity, providing for a great deal of connection and engagement between the child and the adult. This intervention may be especially helpful for children who have a movement-based play preference.

Instructions

1) The practitioner explains to the child that they will be playing a game that requires them to hold hands the entire time.
2) The practitioner stands in one spot and the child stands beside the practitioner.
3) The practitioner takes the child's right hand, and the child starts to walk around the practitioner.
4) As the child gets to the back of the practitioner, the practitioner switches to their left hand and takes the child's right hand as the child continues around the practitioner.
5) The child keeps walking around the practitioner with the practitioner switching hands but always keeping attunement with the child as they walk around the practitioner.
6) After several times of walking around, the practitioner can have the child switch directions and walk around the practitioner in the opposite direction.
7) The practitioner can also have the child walk around them in a specific style such as in slow motion, fast, hopping, skipping, or walking backward.
8) The play continues until the practitioner and child are no longer interested.

Rationale

The Ring Around Me intervention helps children work on connection and relationship development, especially in attuning to another person, making physical connection, and following another person's instructions. It is done through a movement-based play game that provides fun for the child and can help decrease any anxiousness related to interacting with another person. This intervention can be repeated several times and the practitioner and child can switch roles if the child desires. This intervention can be taught to parents to do regularly at home with their child. It can be easily paired with other connection interventions for parent and child to play together at home. Parents can also involve siblings or other family members. Involving other family members to play with the child will likely help generalize relationship and connection development.

Turn Around and Make a Face

Therapy Needs: Connection, relationship development, feeling identification
Level: Child, adolescent
Materials: None
Modality: Individual, family, group

Introduction

This play intervention involves physical movement in a connecting process. It is designed to help children and adolescents work on noticing and connecting with another person. Further, it works on helping children with body awareness and identifying feelings and states of being.

Instructions

1) The practitioner tells the child they are going to play a game where they will be surprising each other with reactions.
2) The practitioner and child stand with their backs to each other. On the practitioner's count of three, the practitioner and child both turn around and create a reaction with their body and face (props can also be used).
3) Each person notices the other person and has to say what kind of reaction they think the other person is displaying.
4) This intervention can be repeated several times; each time the practitioner and child must make a new reaction. The practitioner can also instruct that specific reactions have to be made each time, such as turn around and make a silly face, act bored, feel hunger etc.
5) Play continues until the practitioner and child are no longer interested.

Rationale

This play intervention helps children and adolescents work on connection and relationship development, as well as social navigation and feeling identification and expression. With specific instructions from the practitioner, the child can practice making various reactions that display feelings. This intervention can be taught to parents to do regularly at home with their child. The practitioner should give parents several ideas of reactions to make and practice when completing this intervention with their child at home.

Magnify Me

Therapy Needs: Connection, engagement, relationship development, self-worth
Level: Child

Materials: None
Modality: Individual, family

Introduction

Magnify me is a fun and engaging way for children to work on relationship connection. This intervention helps children interact positively with others, notice others, be comfortable being noticed by others, and to develop a better sense of the child's physical self.

Instructions

1) The practitioner explains to the child that the practitioner will be using a magnifying glass to closely examine different parts of the child.
2) The practitioner uses a toy magnifying glass and looks through the glass, moving over different parts of the child, such as the child's ear, nose, eyes, hair, fingers etc.
3) As the practitioner moves over a part of the child, they should make positive comments such as, 'Wow, you have such a cool nose!' or 'This is some really brown hair.'
4) It is important that the practitioner makes comments about the child and the comments be positive and/or descriptive.
5) The practitioner should then try to get the child to switch roles and have the child look through the magnifying glass at the practitioner. This intervention can be played several times with the practitioner making new comments as they examine the child.

Rationale

This play intervention helps children work on connection and relationship development. Children become more comfortable and aware of their own self and more comfortable with and aware of others. Further, the magnifying glass creates a fun component that also provides a safe distance for the child as they work on engaging. This intervention can be taught to parents to play at home and can be combined with other connection techniques that parents can play with their children regularly between counseling sessions.

Crawling Crabs

Therapy Needs: Connection, engagement, relationship development, attachment
Level: Child
Materials: None
Modality: Individual, family

Introduction

Neurodivergent children may need to work on various connection skills in a way that is less anxiety-producing and more playful and engaging. Crawling Crabs is a simple yet effective connection and touch intervention that helps children (especially young children) develop relationship with others. Further, it helps children understand and become comfortable with positive touch, attuning to another person, and engaging in a mutual process with another person.

Instructions

1) The child sits on the floor with their legs stretched forward and their hands on their legs.
2) The practitioner sits across from the child and starts moving their hands with fingers down on the floor in a walking movement toward the child.
3) When the practitioner reaches the child, the practitioner continues with their hands walking up the child's legs and then up the child's arms until the practitioner reaches the top of the child's arms.
4) At the top of the child's arms, the practitioner gently squeezes the child's shoulders, and the process ends. The practitioner and child can also switch roles if the child desires.
5) The practitioner should explain the game to the child before beginning and complete a demonstration of the touch and movement on a stuffed animal or on the practitioner's own legs and hands.
6) The intervention can be repeated until the practitioner and child are no longer interested.

Rationale

Crawling Crabs helps children work on connection, attachment, and relationship development. This intervention can be taught to parents to do regularly at home with their child. Parents may also combine this intervention with other connection interventions and try to incorporate other family members to play with the child. As with any touch intervention, practitioners and parents should try to be aware of and understand the child's limits in terms of being comfortable with or having a sensory sensitivity to physical touch. Before beginning any intervention that involves touch, practitioners should reference the Association of Play Therapy's paper on touch referenced at the beginning of this book.

Silly Glasses

Therapy Needs: Connection, engagement, relationship development, attachment
Level: Child, adolescent

Materials: Several eye/sunglasses, mirror
Modality: Individual, family, group

Introduction

This play intervention creates a fun process to help children notice and be attuned to themselves and others. There is an interactive component for a child that promotes participating with, connecting, and attachment with others. Joint attention is also a component of this intervention.

Instructions

1) The practitioner explains to the child that they will be playing a game using several different glasses.
2) The practitioner displays several different eye or sunglasses for the child to choose from.
3) The more sunglasses and the more variety of sunglasses that are available will keep the intervention going and make the intervention more interesting to the child.
4) The practitioner explains to the child that they are going to take turns picking out a pair of sunglasses and putting the sunglasses on the other person (it is important that each person choose the sunglasses and place the sunglasses on the other person; the sunglasses should not simply be handed to the other person).
5) Once the sunglasses are in place, the practitioner and child look in a mirror to see themselves in their sunglasses. This process is repeated several times, with the practitioner and child going through several sunglasses.

Rationale

This play intervention helps children work on connection and relationship development, especially in regard to noticing another person and reciprocally interacting with another person. Children also work on attachment and social play with this intervention. This intervention should be taught to parents to do regularly at home with their child. Parents should try to incorporate other family members to play this intervention with the child. Parents will need to collect and have available several types of glasses. Some suggested options for collecting sunglasses would be yard sales and flea markets, where the cost would typically be less.

Hands, Hands, Hands

Therapy Needs: Connection, engagement, sensory regulation, relationship development, attachment
Level: Child, adolescent

Materials: None
Modality: Individual, family, group

Introduction

Sensory-different and other neurodivergent children can have sensory issues with physical touch. They can also experience uncertainty and anxiety when interacting with others. This play intervention provides a simple and fun way to engage with children through a variety of physical touch activities that are presented in play form. The practitioner can engage the child in several hand activities and the intervention can easily be modified to fit the child's comfort level.

Instructions

1) The practitioner explains to the child that they are going to play several games connecting with their hands.
2) The practitioner instructs the child to trace around their hand on a piece of paper.
3) The practitioner then instructs the child to write on the traced hand all the positive things they can think of to do with their hands that involve physically connecting to another person.
4) Once the child is finished, the practitioner can add to the list if the practitioner can think of other positive things.
5) The practitioner and child then do or pretend to do all the things on the list. The practitioner also discusses with the child how connecting with others can be positive, fun, and feel good.
6) The plan continues until the practitioner and child are no longer interested.

Rationale

This play intervention helps children and adolescents work on connection, relationship development, attachment, and sensory regulation. Children learn several positive ways (that are playful and feel good to the child) that they can connect with others through physical touch games. During the intervention, the practitioner should discuss with the child how interacting with others can feel good and be a positive experience. This intervention can be taught to parents to do regularly at home with their child. Parents may need help in coming up with several positive things to do with hands so the practitioner should provide a list of examples for the parents. Some examples include thumb wrestle, high five, hand massage, patty cake, hold hands, creating a special handshake, hand stack game, intertwining fingers, fist pump, lotion hands, pretend palm reading, drawing on person's palm with your finger, arm wrestle, washing hands, palm press, dancing, hand slap (grab) game, and pinky swear.

Sculpture

Therapy Needs: Connection, relationship development, attachment
Level: Child, adolescent
Materials: None
Modality: Individual, family

Introduction

Sculpture connects the child and practitioner together in a way that each person must attune to the other. It also incorporates a physical component that helps with connection between child and practitioner. Children can work on becoming more comfortable with physical touch and interacting with others while engaging in a playful activity.

Instructions

1) The practitioner instructs the child that they are going to take turns making each other into sculptures.
2) The practitioner goes first and moves the child into whatever position they need the child to be in for making the child into a sculpture of something.
3) The practitioner should physically move the child into position by touching the child's arms, legs, etc. and moving them into position, not simply using verbal commands. The child should be sculpted into something real that the child can recognize.
4) Once the child has been made into a sculpture, the child must guess what they have been made into. If the child is struggling to guess, the practitioner can provide hints.
5) The practitioner and child then switch roles and the child gets to make the practitioner into a sculpture of something.
6) This intervention can be repeated several times with the practitioner and child taking turns at making each other into several different sculptures.

Rationale

This play intervention helps children and adolescents work on connection and relationship development, especially interaction with another person and participating in physical touch. It is important that physical touch be included by having the person creating the sculpture physically move the other person into the positions, not just giving verbal instructions. As with any physical touch intervention, the child should have the touch explained and should provide consent. The practitioner will want to make sure that the child is comfortable with the level of physical touch involved. The intervention can be implemented as a family play therapy approach and taught to parents to do at home regularly with their child and the entire family can play together.

Aluminum Wrap

Therapy Needs: Connection, engagement, relationship development, sensory needs, attachment
Level: Child
Materials: Aluminum foil
Modality: Individual, family

Introduction

This play intervention works on both sensory processing and being present with and connecting with another person. It also provides a reciprocal component that is beneficial for relationship development. Aluminum foil is typically used but if the child is uncomfortable with the foil, another similar material could be used.

Instructions

1) The practitioner explains to the child that they are going to use aluminum foil to wrap different parts of their bodies.
2) The practitioner begins by wrapping one of the child's hands in aluminum foil and pressing lightly on the aluminum foil so it molds around the child's hand.
3) The practitioner then takes the aluminum foil off the child's hand and wraps the child's other hand.
4) The practitioner can wrap the child's feet, ears, fingers, anything that would be appropriate but only one body part at a time.
5) The practitioner should notice the child's reaction and be sensitive to the child as each body part is wrapped.
6) The practitioner should ask the child how it feels when one of their body parts is wrapped in aluminum foil.
7) The practitioner should try to engage the child in switching roles and having the child wrap the practitioner's hands and feet in aluminum foil. The child may prefer one role over the other, but it is important to have the child switch roles and be in both positions: being wrapped and wrapping.
8) Once the practitioner and child are finished wrapping each other with aluminum foil, the aluminum foil should be used to make something for each other that the other person can wear on themselves, such as a hat or bracelet.

Rationale

This play intervention helps children work on connection and relationship development. It also works on sensory tactile and touch issues and physical pressure. This intervention can be repeated session to session. It can also be taught to parents to do at home with their child.

Silhouette

Therapy Needs: Connection, engagement, relationship development, attachment	
Level: Child	
Materials: White paper, pencil	
Modality: Individual, family	

Introduction

This play intervention provides the opportunity for the practitioner to connect with the child and the child to attune to and reciprocate back to the practitioner, The intervention creates a visual representation of connection. Silhouette can be simplified or made more complex, depending on the comfort level and age of the child.

Instructions

1) The practitioner explains to the child that they will be using paper and pencils to trace different body parts.
2) The practitioner has the child lay their head down sideways on a white piece of paper. The practitioner traces around the child's head.
3) The child then draws their features on the tracing.
4) The child then traces the practitioner's head while the practitioner lays their head down on a white piece of paper.
5) The practitioner and child then trace each other's hands and lastly feet (if appropriate and the practitioner and child are both comfortable with tracing feet).
6) The traced hands and feet can be colored and decorated by the child.
7) If the practitioner has a large enough piece of paper, the child can lie on the paper and have their whole body traced.
8) The practitioner should try to get the child to reciprocate and trace the practitioner. If the child is not willing to do this, the practitioner should just trace the child.
9) The intervention ends once all the tracing has been completed. The child can keep the tracings as a reminder of the positive connecting experience.

Rationale

This play intervention helps children and adolescents work on connection and relationship development. The practitioner should introduce the intervention to the child so the child understands they will be tracing each other's head, hands, and feet on a white piece of paper. The practitioner will want to ensure that the child is comfortable with the intervention before beginning. This intervention can be taught to parents to do at home with their child.

Family Spin

Therapy Needs: Connection, engagement, relationship development, sensory needs
Level: Child, adolescent
Materials: None
Modality: Individual, family, group

Introduction

This play intervention is typically completed as a family play activity. It can be completed with just the practitioner and child, but tends to work better with a family or in a group setting. It provides an opportunity for family members to connect and engage in a playful game that works on connection and relationship development. It can also provide a sensory-regulating experience for sensory-different children.

Instructions

1) The practitioner instructs the family to make a circle and each family member to put both of their hands in the circle (out in front of them) and everyone grab someone else's hands.
2) Each family member should be holding another family member's hand so the whole family is connected.
3) The practitioner then instructs the family that they will start spinning around to the right slowly.
4) After a period of time, the practitioner will interject various instructions for the family to do such as: speed up, walk in slow motion, start spinning to the left, stop, jump, hop to the right, etc. Types of moves that may be sensory-regulating for sensory-different children can also be included.
5) The practitioner can also play this game with a child one-on-one, and the practitioner and child can take turns being the person who gives the instructions.

6) If the family plays this game at home, one person can be designated as the person who will give the family instructions on how to spin. Each family member can have a turn in this position.
7) The play continues until the family members no longer want to play.

Rationale

This play intervention helps children and adolescents work on connection and relationship development, attuning to others, and physical touch. This intervention is a family intervention and can be done with one parent and one child, or multiple family members. It can also be implemented in a group format. The size does not matter as long as there are at least two people. When the family does the intervention at home, it is helpful if there is one person who stays on the outside of the circle calling out the instructions. If there is no one to do this, then the parent should interject the instructions as they play with the child.

Our Unique Greeting

Therapy Needs: Connection, engagement, relationship development, attachment, social navigation
Level: Child, adolescent
Materials: None
Modality: Individual, family, group

Introduction

Neurodivergent children may feel uncomfortable with meeting and greeting new people. This play intervention provides the opportunity for the practitioner to create a unique greeting with the child or adolescent that can involve many elements but should involve some physical touch. This intervention also helps with social anxiety and connection.

Instructions

1) The practitioner explains to the child that they will be creating a unique greeting they can do each time they see each other. Hands, gestures, and words can all be used in creating the greeting.
2) The practitioner and child can use their unique greeting each time the child comes in for a session. The practitioner and child can also create a unique way to say goodbye at the end of each session.
3) The greeting and/or goodbye should involve some form of physical touch.
4) The practitioner should allow the child to try and come up with the greeting and goodbye on their own. The practitioner should assist the child as needed.

5) Once the practitioner and child have created their unique greeting and goodbye, the practitioner and child should practice the greeting and goodbye several times and plan to use it in the future. If the practitioner creates these with multiple children, the practitioner may want to write down the child's unique greeting in their notes to remember how it is completed.

Rationale

This play intervention helps children and adolescents work on connection and relationship development in the areas of physical touch, acknowledging and attuning to another person, and creating special meaning in a relationship. Once the special greeting and/or goodbye have been created and practiced, the practitioner will want to make sure they remember them so the next time they see the child, the special greeting and goodbye can be implemented. This intervention can be taught to parents to do at home with their child. Each parent, and other family members if appropriate, can all create unique greeting and goodbye rituals with the child.

Together Balloons

Therapy Needs: Connection, engagement, relationship development, social navigation, regulation
Level: Child, adolescent
Materials: Balloon
Modality: Individual, family, group

Introduction

Together Balloons helps address connecting with others and working with and cooperating with others to complete a task. This intervention is designed to be a fun and engaging way for the practitioner and child to work on connection. It also incorporates a social navigation component requiring the practitioner and child to work as a team to complete the task. The practitioner should make sure the child is not afraid of balloons and has no balloon allergies.

Instructions

1) The practitioner explains to the child that they will be playing a game together that involves using a balloon.
2) The practitioner blows up a balloon and ties it off. The practitioner explains to the child that they are going to work together in a special way to keep the balloon in the air.

3) The practitioner and child stand facing each other and grab each other's hands and hold both hands.
4) The practitioner hits the balloon in the air and the practitioner and child must keep the balloon from touching the ground.
5) The practitioner and child maintain holding hands the whole time and move around together to keep the balloon in the air.
6) If the balloon hits the ground, it should be picked up and the game starts again. The game can be repeated several times and played until the practitioner and child are no longer interested.

Rationale

This play intervention helps children and adolescents work on connection and relationship development through physical touch, working cooperatively, and attuning to and being aware of others. Together balloons can be taught to parents to do at home regularly with their child. Other family members can also get involved and play with the child. This intervention works well as a family play activity and a group activity. In a family or group setting, the participants can pair up or function as one large group, holding each other's hands.

Hide and Find

Therapy Needs: Connection, engagement, relationship development
Level: Child, adolescent
Materials: Index cards, pencil
Modality: Individual, family

Introduction

This play intervention addresses therapy goals for children who have challenges in establishing relationships and meaningful connection with others. This intervention provides several opportunities for the child or adolescent to practice relationship and connection. A variety of other needs can be easily incorporated in this intervention such as social navigation, regulation, and feelings identification.

Instructions

1) The practitioner tells the child they are going to play a game where the child is going to find some things the practitioner hides in the room.
2) The practitioner writes various connection activities on index cards and hides the index cards around the playroom (the child should be waiting outside the playroom door or standing in a corner and not watching).

3) Once the practitioner has finished hiding the cards, the child then enters the playroom and has to find all the index cards.
4) When the child finds an index card, they and the practitioner must do the activity that is written on the index card.
5) The practitioner should create around 5–7 index cards. Connection activities should be short and simple. Some examples include shaking hands, giving a double high five, giving a pat on the back, thumb wrestling, etc.
6) The intervention ends once all the cards have been found and all the activities completed.

Rationale

This play intervention helps children and adolescents work on connection and relationship development through a variety of methods. The practitioner can write any connection-related activity on an index card. The practitioner can also include activities that work on improving social navigation needs and feelings identification. The intervention should be taught to parents to do at home. Parents will likely need to be given several ideas for connection activities that can be written on index cards. Parents will need to prepare several index cards and play the intervention using around seven cards; they can play the intervention several times creating a new set of index cards/connection activities each time they play.

Squiggle Drawing Gift

(Adapted from Donald Winnicott's Squiggle Technique)

Therapy Needs: Connection, engagement, relationship development, social navigation
Level: Child, adolescent
Materials: White paper, pencil
Modality: Individual, family, group

Introduction

Neurodivergent children often want to be connected to important people in their lives but can struggle with the process due to anxiety, past rejections, and non-affirming experiences. This play intervention provides the opportunity to work on connection with another person (completing a task together), and it creates a strong visual element to help reinforce learning and remembering the connection. It also presents the opportunity for both people to show each other they are thinking about them and acknowledging them in a meaningful way.

Instructions

1) The practitioner explains to the child they will be doing a drawing activity.
2) The practitioner and child each take a piece of white paper and a pencil and sign their name somewhere on the paper.
3) When the practitioner says go, they both start squiggling all over the paper.
4) This lasts about 10 seconds and then the practitioner says stop.
5) The practitioner and child exchange papers and sign their names somewhere on the new paper and attempt to make a drawing out of the other person's squiggle.
6) After the practitioner and child have finished their drawings, they share with each other what they created for each other and then give the drawing to each other as a gift. The practitioner should process that they have created something together and now have a physical representation of their combined work.
7) The practitioner and child can then complete another squiggle drawing gift; there is no limit on the number of times the activity can be played.

Rationale

This play intervention helps children and adolescents work on connection and relationship development though thinking about and creating something for another person. It also provides the opportunity for the child to create something collaboratively and practice giving another person a gift. The practitioner and child can repeat the squiggle drawing intervention several times. Parents should be taught how to do this intervention at home and instructed to play it with their child regularly. This intervention also works well in a group setting, with each participant pairing up and rotating through the group, creating several drawings.

My Measurements

Therapy Needs: Connection, engagement, relationship development, attachment
Level: Child, adolescent
Materials: None
Modality: Individual, family

Introduction

Autistic and other neurodivergent children may need to engage in connecting activities to become more comfortable and confident in relationship connection and attachment. This play intervention is a fun way to promote relationship connection. The practitioner can adjust this intervention to be simple, with one or two measurements conducted, or more complex, conducting several measurements. The adjustment should match the child's age, comfort level, and interest level.

Instructions

1) The practitioner explains to the child that the practitioner is going to conduct several measurements of the child.
2) Before beginning, the practitioner should give the child an example such as, 'I am going to measure the length of your arm.' The practitioner should then demonstrate the measuring on the practitioner's own arm. The practitioner would gain consent from the child to continue with the intervention.
3) The practitioner conducts various measurements on the child and writes down the child's measurements on a piece of paper.
4) The practitioner should try to get the child to engage in a reciprocal process by having the child conduct some measurements on the practitioner.
5) Some of the types of measurements can include measuring the child's legs, arms, head, feet, hands, height, ears, smile, nose, hair length, fingers, etc.
6) Once the measurements are complete, the child can keep their My Measurements paper where the practitioner has written down all their measurements.

Rationale

This play intervention helps children work on connection and relationship development, especially in the areas of physical touch, receiving positive attention from another person, and engaging in reciprocal and joint attention processes. A cloth or flexible measuring tape works best for this intervention. The practitioner should try to incorporate fun measurements such as the length of the child's smile and the length of the child's fingers. Making the intervention silly and fun will make the intervention more engaging and comfortable for the child. Parents should be taught how to do this intervention at home and encouraged to play the intervention regularly with their child at home. Parents can keep track of the measurements and show the child each time the measurements change.

Bubble Tag

Therapy Needs: Connection, engagement, relationship development, social navigation, sensory needs
Level: Child, adolescent
Materials: Bubbles
Modality: Individual, family, group

Introduction

Bubble Tag incorporates two fun and engaging games for children – bubble blowing and playing tag. Connection and relationship development needs, as well as social navigation and sensory awareness, can be addressed in this intervention. Bubble tag works well in individual intervention but is best played in a family or group setting. The practitioner will need a bottle of bubbles for each person who is participating.

Instructions

1) The practitioner explains to the group that they are going to play a game of tag using bubbles.
2) The practitioner decide on 2–4 people (depends on the size of the group) who will blow the bubbles first (taggers). These people will blow bubbles and try to hit (tag) the other people with a bubble. The taggers are encouraged to work together to tag people.
3) The other people should move around the room and try to avoid getting hit by any bubbles.
4) Once a person is hit by a bubble, they get a bottle of bubbles and join the taggers.
5) The game continues in this way until all participants have been tagged.
6) The game can be lengthened by requiring a person to be tagged by a certain number of bubbles, such as ten bubbles have to hit the person before they become a tagger.
7) This intervention should be played in a room or outdoor setting where the space is somewhat restricted but large enough to move around. Playing in a space that is too small or too large can make it very challenging to enjoy and complete the game.

Rationale

This play intervention helps children work on connection and relationship development skills, as well as social navigation and group play. The children may prefer to stay in one role such as the bubble blower, but the practitioner should encourage the children to switch roles, as each role addresses different need areas. Parents can be taught to implement this intervention at home and encouraged to play with their child. The whole family would participate and play with one bubble blower or assign multiple family members as bubble blowers, working together to tag the rest of the family.

Flower, Rain, and Sun

Therapy Needs: Connection, engagement, relationship development, attachment	
Level: Child	

Materials: None
Modality: Individual, family

Introduction

Feeling comfortable and confident attuning to and playing with another person can be challenging for some neurodivergent children. This play intervention promotes connection and relationship development, as well as joint attention, attachment, and play with another person. Flower, Rain, and Sun also promotes increasing comfort with physical touch and sensory processing. It is a quick, easy, and fun intervention to implement with children.

Instructions

1) The practitioner explains to the child that they will be playing a game that involves some physical touch.
2) The practitioner may want to complete a demonstration on a stuffed animal before implementing the intervention with the child so the child is prepared for what will be happening.
3) The practitioner begins by making a fist and telling the child that the fist is a flower that wants to grow. The flower needs sun and needs to be watered.
4) The child should pretend to give the flower water and sun. The practitioner then slowly opens their fist and spreads their fingers out, representing the flower blooming.
5) The practitioner tells the child that they can smell the flower, touch or feel the flower, or pretend to pick a petal from the flower.
6) The practitioner then pretends to be a snapping flower and when the child touches or smells the flower, the practitioner will gently close their hand on the child's finger or nose.
7) The practitioner and child can play the intervention several times, growing several new flowers. The practitioner and child can also switch roles and the child can pretend to make a flower.
8) The practitioner will want to make sure they explain the game to the child before they begin so the child is not startled by the practitioner implementing the snapping flower component. If the child is uncomfortable with this element, it can be left out of the intervention.

Rationale

This play intervention helps children work on connection and relationship development, especially regarding attuning to another person, participating in a reciprocal activity, and being comfortable with physical proximity and touch. Parents can be taught to play this intervention with their child. This intervention can be implemented with several other connection interventions, as most connection interventions will not require much time to complete.

Hello Friend

(Adapted from Louise Goldberg's Creative Relaxation®)

Therapy Needs: Connection, engagement, relationship development, social navigation
Level: Child, adolescent
Materials: None
Modality: Group, family

Introduction

This intervention is implemented in a family or group setting. Hello friend is a variation of a namaste greeting in the creative relaxation program. This intervention promotes connection and relationship development, as well as attunement, following instructions, and social navigation elements.

Instructions

1) The practitioner explains to the family or group that they will be implementing a special greeting to each other that will be done in a unique format.
2) The family or group will form two circles, an inside circle and an outside circle. The outside circle will be facing the people in the inside circle and conversely the inside circle will be facing the people in the outside circle.
3) Each person will begin by holding the hands of the person in front of them, so a person in the inside circle will reach forward and hold hands with a person in the outside circle.
4) Once everyone is holding someone else's hands, each person will great the other by saying 'Hello friend' three times to the tune of *Three Blind Mice*. Once Hello friend has been said three times, the outside circle shifts to the right and now each person is facing a new person.
5) They again hold hands and say 'Hello friend' three times to the tune of *Three Blind Mice*. This continues until the outside circle has shifted back to their original people.

Rationale

This play intervention helps children work on connection and relationship development, as well as social navigation, especially in the areas of physical touch, attuning to other people, working as a group to accomplish a task, greeting another person, and group peer play. This intervention works best with a larger number of people, and is typically recommended for a family or group with at least five members.

12 Executive Functioning Interventions

Ball Pass

Therapy Needs: Executive functioning needs, relationship development
Level: Child, adolescent
Materials: Small soft ball
Modality: Individual, group

Introduction

ADHD and other neurodivergent children and adolescents may have needs related to executive functioning. This play intervention presents a simple game play that can help children practice focus, concentration, and whole-brain activation (multi-tasking), specifically listening, asking questions, and monitoring the amount of time to talk about a subject. It is also a fun social interaction relationship-building intervention.

Instructions

1) The practitioner gives instruction to the child that they are going to pass a soft ball back and as they do this, they will need to be naming something in a rhythm with tossing the ball back and forth.
2) The practitioner and child will agree upon a subject. Some examples would be things I see in the room, things that start with the first letter of my name, things I can hear right now, things I notice about the other person.
3) The subject is chosen, and the ball is tossed back and forth, and the person must say something from the subject within two seconds of catching the ball and throwing it back to the other person.
4) If someone messes up, the game starts over, and a new subject can be chosen.
5) Play continues until the practitioner and child are no longer interested.

DOI: 10.4324/9781003398691-12

Rationale

Neurodivergent children may need help with executive functioning areas and addressing these needs through a play process can be helpful for the child to process, retain, and feel good about what they have accomplished. Ball Pass helps children and adolescents work on executive functioning needs and connecting with another person through a simple ball tossing format. Parents can be taught this intervention and should practice at home with their child. If appropriate, parents could involve siblings or other family members in group play.

Take it to the Judge

Therapy Needs: Executive functioning needs, social navigation, self-worth
Level: Child, adolescent
Materials: None
Modality: Individual, group

Introduction

Neurodivergent children and adolescents often have thoughts and beliefs about themselves and the world around them that are not accurate and can produce anxiety, depression, and low self-worth. Many of these beliefs are driven by ableist and non-valuing (non-affirming) messages from other sources and people. Take it to the Judge is an intervention that helps adolescents challenge their inaccurate thoughts and beliefs while working on various executive functioning skills.

Instructions

1) This intervention is often implemented after the practitioner has gotten to know the child or adolescent well and has conceptualized several of the inaccurate beliefs the child might be having.
2) The practitioner makes a list of some of the inaccurate thoughts and presents the list to the child.
3) The child chooses one to begin with. The practitioner explains they are going to take this thought to the 'Judge' who will be played by the practitioner.
4) The child will be the attorney for both sides, arguing to the judge why the thought is accurate and arguing to the judge why the thought is not accurate.
5) The child is given a few minutes to prepare what they want to say (their arguments for both sides).

6) The child then presents both sides to the practitioner. The practitioner addresses what is presented and makes a verdict. The practitioner might also ask for more proof or information for one or both sides or may introduce new evidence into the case.
7) Once the final verdict is given, the practitioner should process with the child why the decision was made and help the child see a new awareness.

Rationale

This play intervention can help children with organizing of thought processes, can improve self-worth, and dispel negative, inaccurate views of self. The practitioner will want to use rational, concrete information to help the child see any inaccurate thoughts. The process can be repeated for any identified inaccurate thoughts until all have been addressed.

Make Me Look

Therapy Needs: Executive functioning needs, connection, relationship development
Level: Child, adolescent
Materials: None
Modality: Individual, family, group

Introduction

This intervention helps children and adolescents learn to be more comfortable in engaging with another person. It also assists with executive functioning needs related to body awareness and focus/concentration. Affirming note: The practitioner should be sensitive to the child's possible anxiety and discomfort in interacting with others when implementing this intervention.

Instructions

1) The practitioner instructs the child that the practitioner is going to stand or sit in one spot and the child can move all around, trying to get the practitioner to notice them.
2) The child can move around, make faces, act silly, tell jokes, pretty much anything goes! The limit should be given that the child cannot touch the practitioner or throw anything at the practitioner.
3) After a few minutes, the practitioner and child should switch roles, so the child is trying to stay focused and not notice the practitioner. The practitioner will try to move around, make noises, make silly faces to try to get the child to notice them.

4) This intervention should be silly and fun. If someone does notice the other person, they can refresh and start over. The game can be continued until the practitioner and child are no longer interested.

Rationale

Make Me Notice helps children work on connection and focus and concentration skills. This intervention can be played several times for any length of time. The practitioner and child should switch roles back and forth. When the practitioner is still, the child is working on noticing the practitioner and creating ideas to get attention. When the child is still, the child is working on body awareness, impulse control, and focus/concentration.

Instruction Puzzle

Therapy Needs: Executive functioning
Level: Child, adolescent
Materials: Small blank puzzle, markers
Modality: Individual, group

Introduction

Visual aids can be helpful for many neurodivergent children. Instruction Puzzle provides an engaging way to create a visual task schedule for children and adolescents. The puzzle pieces serve as steps to complete, and the puzzle can be completed as the child accomplishes each of the steps. The practitioner will need to provide a small, blank puzzle – typically six to nine pieces.

Instructions

1) The practitioner will give the child a small, blank puzzle, typically six pieces for a young child and nine for an adolescent. Blank puzzles can be found online through many education supply stores.
2) The practitioner and child will write instructions, on the front of each puzzle piece, broken down in steps, toward completing something.
3) The practitioner and child will decide on something the child wants to complete, such as how to create a Facebook account, steps to brushing your teeth, morning routine, or how to check out a book at the library (a task or activity should be chosen that the child needs help with or does not know how to do).
4) The child will try to write on the front of each puzzle piece (going in order) steps to accomplish or complete the task. The child can also add pictures to describe each step or just draw pictures without any words.

5) The practitioner should allow the child to complete as much of the instruction puzzle as they can, and the practitioner can assist the child as needed.
6) Once the instructions/steps have been written on all the puzzle pieces and the instructions are complete, the practitioner and child put the puzzle together in the appropriate order for each step to complete the task.
7) The practitioner and child take turns picking a piece of the puzzle and explain or teach that instruction to the other person until the whole puzzle is complete. The practitioner and child can practice completing the task several times.
8) The child can take the puzzle home and use it as a visual aid to help complete the identified task or process.

Rationale

This play intervention it designed as a visual aid to help children and adolescents work on task completion and giving instructions to others. It also serves as a visual task completing tool for the child, as the child and parents could use this format for other tasks. Several puzzles can be made to address several different processes. Figure 12.1 provides an example of a completed puzzle.

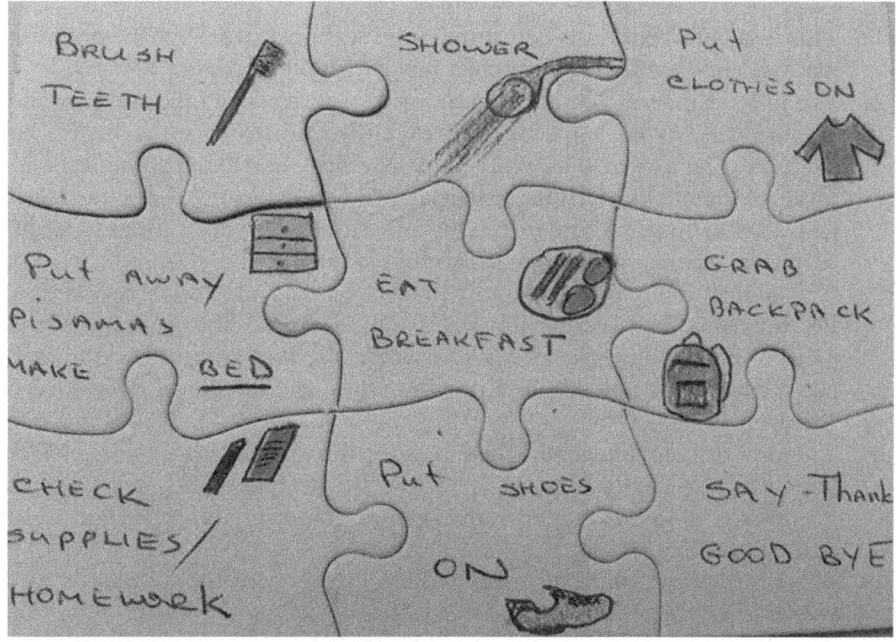

Figure 12.1 Instruction puzzle example.

Robert Jason Grant

Executive Functioning Postcards

Therapy Needs: Executive functioning needs, strengths development, advocacy
Level: Child, adolescent
Materials: Postcards, pencil
Modality: Individual, group

Introduction

ADHD and other neurodivergent children and adolescents may struggle with some executive functioning needs and typically have executive function strengths. This play intervention uses postcard writing play to help the child understand their needs and strengths. The practitioner will want to provide several postcards for the child to choose from when implementing the intervention. Executive functioning skills include self-restraint, working memory, emotion control, focus, task initiation, planning/prioritization, organization, time management, defining and achieving goals, flexibility, observation, perseverance, and stress tolerance.

Instructions

1) This play intervention is best done using real postcards, but the practitioner and child can make their own postcards out of paper.
2) The practitioner and child begin by writing postcards to the child reminding the child what some of their executive functioning needs are. For example, one postcard may say 'Dear Me, remember that sometimes it is hard to remember multiple tasks given to you all at once.' The postcards can also include pictures that the practitioner or child draws, if that would be more appropriate or helpful for the child.
3) The practitioner and child can make as many executive functioning needs postcards as is relevant for the child. An additional element that can be included on the needs postcards is a line about how the child can advocate for their need or what they should do to take care of themselves.
4) The practitioner and child then create postcards identifying the child's strengths, especially around executive functioning. The postcards are written in the same manner as the needs cards, reminding the child about their strength.
5) The practitioner and child can write as many strength postcards as is relevant for the child.
6) The child is instructed to take the postcards home and keep them accessible so they can remember their needs, how to take care of their needs, and all the strengths they possess.

Rationale

The Executive Functioning Postcards intervention provides children and adolescents with a visual aid that they can keep and refer to help them remember their executive functioning self – needs and strengths. It also addresses advocacy or strategies the child can implement to help with executive functioning needs. Parents can be taught this intervention and encouraged to review the postcards with their child at home.

Example postcard statements

'Dear Me, remember that you may forget part of a process or instruction. It is okay to start over, ask for clarification and reset.'

'Dear Me, remember that you can organize anything! You organize LEGO® bricks all the time and have all your Pokémon cards organized. This is a strength you have.'

Fishy and Shark

Therapy Needs: Executive functioning needs, connection, relationship development, attachment
Level: Child
Materials: None
Modality: Individual, family

Introduction

Playing with another person, paying attention to others, and engaging in physical contact with another person can be dysregulating and anxiety-producing areas for neurodivergent children. This play intervention utilizes a simple hand game to help children work on enjoying and feeling regulated in playful and engaging processes with others.

Instructions

1) Fishy and Shark is a hand game that is done between the practitioner and the child.
2) The practitioner and child sit on the floor across from each other but close enough to touch.
3) The child could also sit on a chair with the practitioner on the floor or they could both sit at a table.
4) The practitioner puts their hands together and moves them across the floor wiggling them like a fish swimming. The practitioner wiggles their hands toward the child saying, 'Fishy, fishy.'

5) When the practitioner gets close to the child, the child says, 'Shark,' and takes their hands and clamps down on the practitioner's hands which are making the fish.
6) The process is then reversed with the child being the Fishy and the practitioner being the Shark.
7) Play continues until the practitioner and child no longer want to play.
8) If the concept of a Fishy and Shark is scary or triggering for the child, the practitioner can make it nondescript, saying 'moving hands' and clamping hands' or anything else they can think of to label the hands.

Rationale

Fishy and Shark helps children work on connection and relationship development, especially in attuning to and enjoying play with another person. This play intervention also incorporates increasing concentration, impulse control, and shared attention. Fishy and Shark can be taught to parents, and parents should be encouraged to play this intervention with their children regularly at home. This intervention can be included with other connection interventions, so parents can play several connection interventions during one playtime. Parents can also try to incorporate other family members to play this intervention with the child.

What Am I?

Therapy Needs: Executive functioning, deductive reasoning, social navigation, asking questions
Level: Child, adolescent
Materials: Index cards, tape, pencil
Modality: Individual, family, group

Introduction

Neurodivergent children may struggle with feeling comfortable interacting with another person and asking questions. Often children can have various executive functioning needs. This play intervention helps children and adolescents work on asking other people questions, maintaining focus and attention, and deductive reasoning/organization. This intervention is adapted from the boardgame Hedbanz.

Instructions

1) The practitioner explains to the child that they will be playing a card guessing game.
2) On index cards, the practitioner and child (if the child wants) write several different things such as types of food, animals, toys, material objects,

etc. There should be a variety of items and one item is written on each index card (the cards could be created prior to the child coming in for a session).

3) The index cards should be placed on the floor with the written-on side face down.

4) The practitioner and child each choose one card and put a small piece of tape on the blank side and tape the card to their chest without looking at what is written on it.

5) The practitioner and child then take turns asking the other questions to try and discover what is written on the index card taped on their chest.

6) The practitioner and child cannot look down at what is written on the index card taped to their chest.

7) When someone accurately guesses what is written on their index card, they can put tape on another card and continue with the process until all the cards have been guessed or the practitioner and child no longer want to play the intervention.

Rationale

This playful game provides the opportunity to address needs in a way that decreases possible anxiety and provides enjoyment for the child. This play intervention is designed to help children and adolescents practice and strengthen some executive functioning needs, become more comfortable asking questions, and improve relationship development.

Break Out

Therapy Needs: Executive functioning needs, sensory needs
Level: Child, adolescent
Materials: Toilet paper or crepe paper
Modality: Individual, family, group

Introduction

The Break Out play intervention helps children and adolescents attune to impulse control and be aware of their own physical self. Further, it promotes a sensory-based experience that ADHD, sensory-different and other neurodivergent children may find regulating.

Instructions

1) The practitioner explains to the child that the practitioner is going to wrap the child's legs and arms in crepe paper (toilet paper can also be used) and the child is going to bust out of the wrapping.

2)   The practitioner begins by wrapping one part of the child's body such as the child's legs in toilet paper or crepe paper. The practitioner should wrap around multiple times but not so much that the child cannot break out.

3)   The child is instructed to remain still until the practitioner has finished wrapping the child's legs. Once the practitioner has finished, the practitioner says, 'I will count down slowly, 3, 2, 1 and then say "Go!"'

4)   The child breaks out of the wrapping.

5)   The practitioner then wraps another part of the child's body such as their arms and repeats the process.

6)   The practitioner can also wrap the child's hands and the child's entire body. If the child wants, the practitioner and child can switch roles and the child can wrap the practitioner.

7)   Play continues until the child no longer wants to play.

Rationale

Break Out helps children and adolescents work on impulse control, body awareness, and sensory regulation. It also works on attuning to another person and interoceptive issues. This intervention should be repeated several times. This intervention can be taught to parents to do at home with their child. Parents should be encouraged to make the intervention fun and animated and switch roles with the child, letting the child wrap the parent. Parents can even include the entire family in the intervention.

My Island

(Contributed by Jessica Stone Registered Play Therapist Supervisor™)

Therapy Needs: Flexibility of approach (i.e.,there is not only one way to achieve something, and the ways are still defined)
Level: Child, adolescent
Materials: Nintendo Switch or Lite, Animal Crossing software; Nintendo online access if using two devices and visiting each other's islands
Modality: Individual, family, group

Introduction

Animal Crossing New Horizons is a single- or multi-player game available only for the Nintendo Switch handheld console device. This game has been described as a 'community simulation video game series developed and published by Nintendo, in which the human player (main player) lives in a village inhabited by anthropomorphic animals, carrying out various activities including fishing, bug catching, fossil hunting, etc.' (Fandom, n. d. a, para. 1).

Game play includes a main character (the human player) and up to ten village residents who live on the island with the player. Development of the island, the main character's home, relationships with the village residents, and more activities, goals, and features are defined within the parameters of the game, but are not required by the game play. Daily tasks can be completed if desired and the main player can customize the island to meet their desires, style, and needs.

Animal Crossing New Horizons islands are as unique as the main player. There are simultaneous feelings of control and escape and structure and freedom within the game play. The island is the player's domain, to decorate, populate, and change as desired. As stated by Stone (2022),

> 'In times of chaos and feelings of a lack of predictability in one's real-world environment, it is a re-centering escape to have experiences of mastery and control. This game has limitations and typically will not attract an action-oriented gamer, but for some it is the perfect pace.'
>
> (p. 236)

Cognitive flexibility, or flexibility in thinking, includes the ability to think about multiple things at once, switching between cognitive tasks quickly, and thinking about something in multiple ways simultaneously. As one of several important executive functioning tasks, cognitive flexibility is important in our day-to-day tasks, interactions, understandings, behaviors, and experiences.

Researchers postulate that two types of neurodivergence, Autistic and attention deficit hyperactivity disorder (ADHD), both have elements of difference in cognitive flexibility. 'While Autistic is characterized by difficulty in flexibly adapting to changes in routines, children with ADHD have difficulty with attentional focus and exhibit high levels of variability in moment-to-moment behaviors' (Uddin, 2021, p. 173). Understanding the way one's level of cognitive flexibility creates needs can be critical within therapeutic goals. Finding ways to improve aspects of these flexibilities can greatly improve a person's day-to-day experience (World Economic Forum, 2023). This Digital Play Therapy™ intervention allows the user to practice components of cognitive flexibility within defined parameters throughout the game play.

Instructions

1) The practitioner has assessed the child and determined if any difficulties with cognitive flexibility are present.
2) The practitioner and child have determined the availability of the hardware and software necessary to complete the intervention.
3) The practitioner and child have determined if there is motivation to play the game Animal Crossing New Horizons.

4) The practitioner can employ Level 2 Digital Play Therapy and watch and witness the play while the child plays the game.

    a. The practitioner will observe the decision-making process and decisions made within the game play, applying cognitive flexibility needs to the conceptualization of what is witnessed.

    b. The practitioner will comment, ask questions, intervene, and/or become involved as the therapy plan and theoretical foundation dictates.

    c. The practitioner takes note of the task approaches and response patterns employed by the child and looks for congruencies and incongruencies between what is being demonstrated in the game and what happens in day-to-day life.

    d. If the child is too cognitively flexible – leaves tasks which were previously important incomplete, shifts too quickly between aspects, does not attend to the environment, etc. – the clinical goals would include recognition of difficulties this approach leads to within the game play.

    e. If the child lacks cognitive flexibility – perseverates on one task, has difficulty shifting to other aspects, becomes entranced in the environment beyond appreciation and noticing, etc. – the clinical goals would include recognition of difficulties this approach leads to within the game play, and ultimately in day-to-day life. (This could be by example and experience (indirect teaching) or verbally explained (direct teaching) (Schaefer and Drewes, 2014).)

5) The practitioner can employ Level 3 Digital Play Therapy and join in the play with two devices, two games, and the ability to visit each other's islands via Nintendo Online access.

    a. The practitioner will observe the decision-making process and decisions made within the game play, applying cognitive flexibility needs to the conceptualization of what is witnessed.

    b. The practitioner will comment, ask questions, intervene, and/or become involved as the therapy plan and theoretical foundation dictate.

    c. The practitioner takes note of the task approaches and response patterns employed by the child and looks for congruencies and incongruencies between what is being demonstrated in the game and what happens in day-to-day life.

    d. If the child is too cognitively flexible – leaves tasks which were previously important incomplete, shifts too quickly between aspects, does not attend to the environment, etc. – the clinical goals would include recognition of difficulties this approach leads to within the game play.

    e. If the child lacks cognitive flexibility – perseveres on one task, has difficulty shifting to other aspects, becomes entranced in the environment beyond appreciation and noticing, etc. – the clinical goals would include recognition of difficulties this approach leads to within the game play, and ultimately in day-to-day life. (This could be by example and experience (indirect teaching) or verbally explained (direct teaching) (Schaefer and Drewes, 2014).)

Rationale

This play intervention assists clients of all ages with the expansion or restriction of cognitive flexibility. Cognitive flexibility intervention has been shown to restructure thinking toward more flexible options, extract information within complex dynamics, decipher streams of sensory information, improved cognitive tasks, improved social interaction and communication, greater resilience and well-being, and maximize creative innovations and ideas (World Economic Forum, 2021). The use of Animal Crossing New Horizons allows for the simultaneous structure and flexibility to allow for powerful interactions toward healthy cognitive flexibility.

References

Schaefer, C. E. & Drewes, A. (2014). *The therapeutic powers of play: 20 core agents of change*, 2nd ed. Wiley.

Stone, J. (2022). *Digital play therapy: A clinician's guide to comfort and competence*, 2nd ed. Routledge.

Uddin, L. Q. (2021). Cognitive and behavioral flexibility: Neural mechanisms and clinical considerations. *Nature Reviews: Neuroscience*, 22, 167–179.

World Economic Forum (2021, June 25). Why is cognitive flexibility important and how can you improve it? *Weforum.org*. https://www.weforum.org/agenda/2021/06/cognitive-flexibility-thinking-iq-intelligence/

A Shared Story

(Contributed by Nicky Trussler Mental Health Social Worker)

Therapy Needs: Executive functioning, relationship development and connection, emotional regulation
Level: Child, adolescent
Materials: A selection of small toys, objects, pictures (6–12 in total) and a bag/box to put them in
Modality: Family, group

Introduction

This play intervention can work in a number of different ways, depending on the therapeutic goals. The shared story also builds connections and helps relationship development by cooperating in a shared task, taking turns, and mutually having fun. Many neurodivergent children and adolescents find generating story ideas for writing tasks at school very difficult. This can help to build the skill of storytelling in a supportive and structured way. Finally, as no one person is responsible for the whole story, and nobody knows how it will end, this provides an opportunity to support children to enter the unknown in a safe way and co-regulate as needed, especially if the story direction heads in a way that the child is not expecting, or waiting for their turn to participate is difficult.

Instructions

1) The practitioner explains that each participant in turn pulls an item from the bag and uses it as a prompt to start a story, adding a few words to a few minutes of dialogue. Initially the items in the bag can be quite concrete such as a plastic elephant, a dolls house doll's bed, a pencil, a picture of a beach, or an emoji. More abstract items can be added if appropriate, for example, a leaf, a picture of a person with an empty thought bubble, or a rock.

2) When the first person has added their part, the bag is passed onto the next person, who pulls out another item and continues the previous story incorporating the new prompt.

3) The story continues until all the objects have been taken from the bag, with the last person responsible for trying to find a way to end the story.

4) This is an intervention which can be easily replicated at home or anywhere, as there are no 'set' items that are needed. In fact, it is much more fun if they frequently change so new stories can be developed.

5) Additions to this intervention could be continuing a previous story or reusing a previous character to create a series of wacky stories.

6) This intervention can be played between the practitioner and the child but is more dynamic for family and group work.

Rationale

Common therapy goals for neurodivergent children often include developing skills to executive functioning tasks and social navigation needs in relation to turn-taking and listening to others. This play intervention offers scaffolding to support the development of these everyday skills in a safe and contained way, which can be titrated in terms of difficulty, depending on the needs of the child. The child can be provided with a range of different ideas and scenarios that others present throughout the game, which they also need to listen to and understand to enable them to make their own contributions; but there are also no right or wrong answers. The child is not being 'taught' neurotypical 'social skills' but provided with an opportunity to engage with others in a way that is fair and enjoyable for all. This intervention can be most beneficial when repeated at home periodically with a variety of different items.

Hula Hoop Balloons

Therapy Needs: Executive functioning needs, regulation, social navigation	
Level: Child, adolescent	

Materials: Two hula hoops
Modality: Individual, group

Introduction

This play intervention provides a joint hula hoop game that helps children activate their whole brain, increase concentration, improve body awareness, and help with regulation needs. The game is implemented in a fun and silly manner, and the practitioner and child can create their own variations.

Instructions

1) The practitioner provides two hula hoops and explains to the child that they are going to play a game together using the hula hoops.
2) They will work as a team to roll the hula hoops back and forth to each other and try to stay in a rhythm, without any of the hula hoops going astray.
3) Each person will place their hula hoop in their right hand and when the practitioner says 'Go!', they will each roll to the other person who will catch the hula hoop with their left hands. They will then roll the hula hoop back with their left hands and catch with their right hands. This rhythm will continue until one or both hula hoops go astray. If the rhythm is broken, the practitioner and child can simply start again.
4) A variation or switch up of this game would be to toss the hula hoops back and forth and catch them in the air.
5) The intervention is continued until the practitioner and child are no longer interested.

Rationale

Children and adolescents may have needs regarding focus, concertation, and regulation. This play intervention combines elements to address multiple needs (including body awareness and regulation). The hula hoop game format provides strengthening of needs through a fun and engaging play game. The atmosphere of the intervention should be fun and silly. The focus is on attempting the rhythm and continuing attempts, not on mastery.

Do It This Way

Therapy Needs: Executive functioning needs
Level: Child, adolescent
Materials: None
Modality: Individual, group

Introduction

Children and adolescents who need help with executive functioning areas often become stigmatized and negatively mislabeled due to their needs. It is important that children can work on addressing their needs in a play-focused environment without the construct of 'failing'. This play intervention helps address needs such as multi-tasking, memory recall, and hearing instructions.

Instructions

1) The practitioner explains that they are going to play a game where they instruct each other to do certain things in a certain way.
2) The practitioner would go first to provide an example. The practitioner would say something like, 'I want you to put miniature with red on it in the sand tray and I want you to do this acting like a robot'.
3) The practitioner should not repeat the instruction but encourage the child to do what they can remember. The practitioner should remember to keep the instructions fun and silly.
4) Once the child has competed the task, they get to give the practitioner an instruction to complete.
5) Play continues back and for the (taking turns) until the practitioner and child no longer want to play. Some other instruction examples include: draw a square on a piece of paper as an eagle, or make three baskets in the basketball hoop like a person who is really scared.

Rationale

This play intervention is designed to help children hear and recall information for multiple task completion. The intervention is implemented in a fun and silly play format. The atmosphere should be playful and if the child forgets a piece of the instruction, the child should not feel shamed but encouraged for what they did remember. Neurodiversity note: Children and adolescents who work on any executive functioning needs should always be valued and encouraged. They should not be made to feel that they have a deficit, or they are less than or problematic because of how their brain works.

Under Which Cup

Therapy Needs: Executive functioning needs, self-worth
Level: Child, adolescent
Materials: Three small paper cups, one sticker
Modality: Individual, group

Introduction

ADHD and other neurodivergent children may have executive functioning needs in the areas of focus and concentration. This is a simple play intervention that utilizes cups to help the child improve maintaining focus and attention. Small paper cups are the best option, but any type of disposable cup can be used.

Instructions

1) The practitioner explains that they will be playing a game and the child will be concentrating to get the correct answer.
2) The practitioner displays three small paper cups and one of the cups has a sticker on the inside bottom. The practitioner should have placed the sticker prior to the session.
3) The practitioner shows the child the one with the sticker and places all three cups in front of the child and practitioner. This intervention is best completed on a table or a smooth floor surface.
4) The practitioner will move the cups around and the child will try to maintain focus on the cup that has the sticker. After the cups have been moved around a bit, the child will try to guess which cup has the sticker.
5) If the child does not guess correctly, they can try again and this time the practitioner can move the cups a bit more slowly. If the child guesses correctly, they can play again, and the practitioner should move the cups more quickly or for a longer amount of time.
6) The practitioner will want to start by moving the cups slowly and for a short amount of time, and then increase the speed and length of time as the child guesses the correct cups.
7) As the child progresses in guessing the correct cup, the practitioner can add in other distracting elements. This might include opening a window blind so the child can see activity outside the window or playing a video on a smartphone or tablet beside the child while they are focusing on the cups.
8) The play should stay fun and not become frustrating for the child. The practitioner and child can continue to play until they are no longer interested.

Rationale

Children and adolescents may need help in strengthening their focus and concentration. This play game helps children improve these areas of executive functioning and helps them feel more confident in themselves. Often children can receive negative messages about themselves due to executive functioning needs. This intervention can be used to help strengthen the child's self-worth.

What's Different

Therapy Needs: Executive functioning needs
Level: Child, adolescent
Materials: A selection of miniatures or flash cards
Modality: Individual, group

Introduction

This play intervention is designed to help children and adolescents strengthen executive functioning needs in the areas of focus, concentration, and memory recall. The practitioner will need a selection of various miniatures or flash cards.

Instructions

1) The practitioner explains to the child that they will be playing a focusing game using miniatures.
2) The practitioner and child sit facing each other (at a table or on the floor). The practitioner places approximately four to five miniatures in front of the child.
3) The practitioner asks the child to look at the miniatures, noting what they are and their placement. The child can take as much time as they need to notice the miniatures.
4) When the child is ready, the child will turn around and the practitioner will change something about the miniatures. The child will turn back around and try to identify what is different.
5) The practitioner should begin with small changes such as moving one miniature out of order or taking one miniature away. As the child guesses correctly, the practitioner can make the process more challenging by adding more miniatures and making more than one change.
6) The process should remain fun for the child and help increase their confidence in maintaining concentration and memory recall. The goal is to help the child feel successful. The practitioner should move at the child's pace and ensure they are able to make accurate guesses.
7) Play can continue until the practitioner and child are no longer interested.

Rationale

Neurodivergent children with executive functioning needs may require help to strengthen concentration and memory recall. This intervention provides a fun game format to work on this need area. It also allows for the child to experience success and improve their confidence and self-worth.

Balloon Release

Therapy Needs: Executive functioning needs, identity, self-worth	
Level: Child, adolescent	
Materials: Balloon	
Modality: Individual, group	

Introduction

ADHD and other neurodivergent children may have specific ways their brain works. Some children need help understanding and appreciating their brain and differences in the way they operate compared to others. Balloon Release utilizes blowing up and releasing a balloon to help the child better understand how their own brain works and to help them appreciate their identity an individual with ADHD and/or a neurodivergent individual.

Instructions

1) The practitioner explains to the child that they are going to blow up a balloon and then release it. The child is given the instruction to try and catch the balloon before it hits the ground.
2) The practitioner says, 'Go!' and releases the balloon. This process happens very quickly and should be repeated a few times.
3) After a few times, the practitioner explains that they are going to release the balloon and the child needs to try and follow the path the balloon goes. This new process is then repeated a few times.
4) The practitioner and child then take a break and talk about the balloon as an analogy for different brains. The practitioner should explain that the balloon is like different brains. It is fun to blow up the balloon and release it and play different games, but it would also be fun to blow up the balloon and tie it off and play other games. Both ways the balloon can operate are fun and have benefits. This is how brains also work.
5) The practitioner can also discuss with the child how the balloon going all over the place may feel like them and their brain. If the child relates to the release balloon, the practitioner can explain that the release balloon (brain) is a lot of fun and we can do cool things with it, just like the other type of balloon (brain) can be fun and we can do cool things with it.
6) The practitioner and child can process as needed and the child should have the opportunity to ask any questions or make comments. They can continue to play the intervention until they are no longer interested.

Rationale

This play intervention is designed to help children with 'active brains' to better understand themselves in an affirming way. The balloon play provides an experiential example to help the child process. This intervention could be paired with bibliotherapy – reading books about different brains or neurodivergence.

13 Strengths Development Interventions

Hearts In Hands

(Contributed by Danyale Weems, Registered Play Therapist Supervisor™)

Therapy Needs: Strengths development, connection, and relationship development
Level: Child, adolescent
Materials: Pencil, construction paper, paint/colored pencils/markers, scissors, glue, cut-outs of various shapes and sizes of hearts, flashlight, gloves
Modality: Individual, family

Introduction

Parents in the lives of neurodivergent children and adolescents often struggle with connecting and validating the unique qualities that their child possesses. Neurodivergent children and adolescents often struggle to identify and communicate their unique qualities to parents. They may have difficulty recognizing the many supports/helpers in their environment. This play and expressive intervention helps parents and children to connect relationally. It also helps parents and/or their children to identify the child's strengths, providing a strengths-based language for the child's unique differences.

Instructions

1) The practitioner and child cut various heart shapes out of different colors of paper.
2) The child chooses a color of construction paper and the practitioner, using a pencil, traces one of the child's hands on the paper.
3) The child then traces the practitioner's opposite hand, with a pencil, on the same paper, beside the child's hand. When the hands are traced side by side, the thumbs should overlap, forming a heart shape. Figure 13.1 provides a Hearts in Hands example.

DOI: 10.4324/9781003398691-13

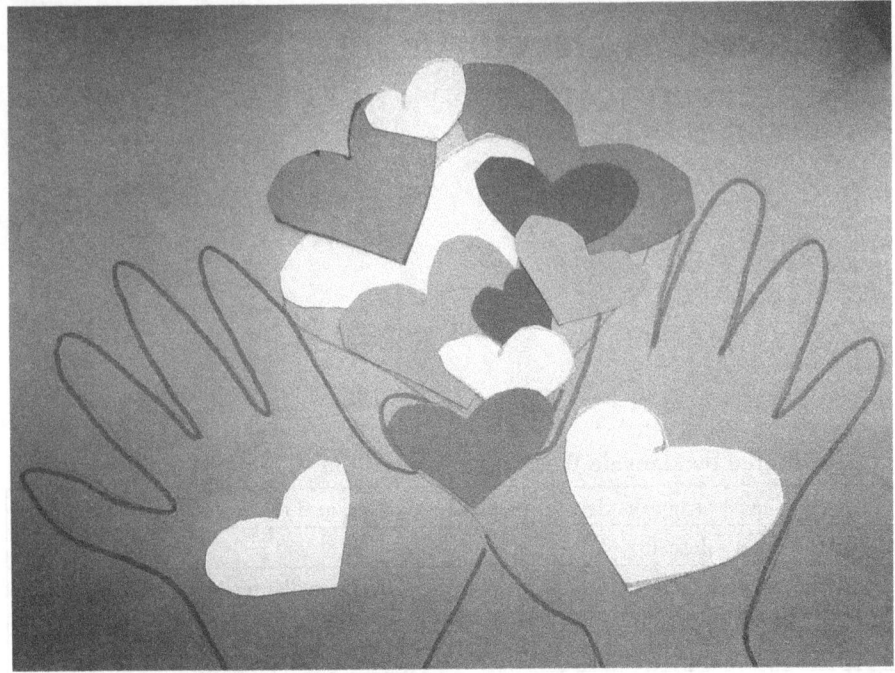

Figure 13.1 Hearts in hands example.

Danyale Weems

4) The practitioner and child then use a marker to trace the outline of both hands including the outline of the thumbs (not where they intersect).
5) The practitioner and child identify various people (friends, relatives, teachers, youth leaders, etc.) and pets who love the child and who the child loves.
6) An alternate version or additional element can focus on strengths. The practitioner and child identify strengths and write them on the hearts (having a list of strengths specific to the child and/or neurodivergent children can be helpful).
7) As the child identifies their strengths, the practitioner should encourage them to give an example of their strength, for example: 'I love how you get excited when you talk about something you love or regulate yourself by rocking back and forth.'

Rationale

This play intervention provides an expressive visual and tactile experience designed to assist the parents and child with connection and relationship development. It is also designed to help provide a voice for the child or adolescent to explore their differences as strengths. This activity helps the parents to view the differences in a positive perspective.

Blegerblag

(Contributed by Sarah Moran Registered Play Therapist Supervisor™)

Therapy Needs: Strengths development, executive functioning, and connection	
Level: Child, adolescent	
Materials: Paper, markers, timer, miscellaneous art supplies (e.g. glue, felt, ribbon, popsicle sticks, googly eyes, gems, beads, feathers, etc.)	
Modality: Individual, family, group	

Introduction

Neurodivergent children and adolescents often have trouble with executive functioning skills, including processing information, planning, organizing, remembering information and details, and staying on topic. This play therapy intervention is a simple game that helps children understand their strengths, and recognize their executive function needs as they create, problem solve, and connect with others to better understand the value of neurodiversity in a creative world. This play intervention can be done simply with pencil and paper, or a variety of art materials.

Instructions

1) The practitioner explains to the child that they will be playing a game where there is no right or wrong way to play, because everyone's brain and imagination is unique. It is common for a child to freeze and/or refuse due to high anxiety in not knowing what to do or perceiving how to do it 'right.' If questions are asked for details, remind them that their brains are creating the answers, and this game can be repeated.
2) The practitioner invites the child to come up with a nonsense word (for example, 'Clarsh') and draw a picture of what it might look like (including vague shape and characteristics). The child is instructed to hide this drawing from the practitioner.
3) The practitioner also works on drawing their nonsense word, 'Blegerblag,' and hides this drawing from the child.
4) The practitioner instructs the child to create a 'Blegerblag' using their chosen art supplies, while the therapist works on creating a 'Clarsh'. It can truly be anything (object, imaginary friend, animal, person, etc.). The practitioner sets a timer for how long they will work on this project (e.g., 15–20 minutes).
5) Typically the practitioner and child will work on their individual projects sitting back-to-back or facing away from each other.
6) Once completed, the therapist asks the child to show their creation of a 'Blegerblag', and the therapist shares their creation of a 'Clarsh'. These

creations are then compared to the original drawing made by the non-sense word creator. The practitioner invites the child to find comparisons between the drawing and art, if there are any (such as: they are both objects, or they both have eyes). Figures 13.2 and 13.3 demonstrate completed examples.

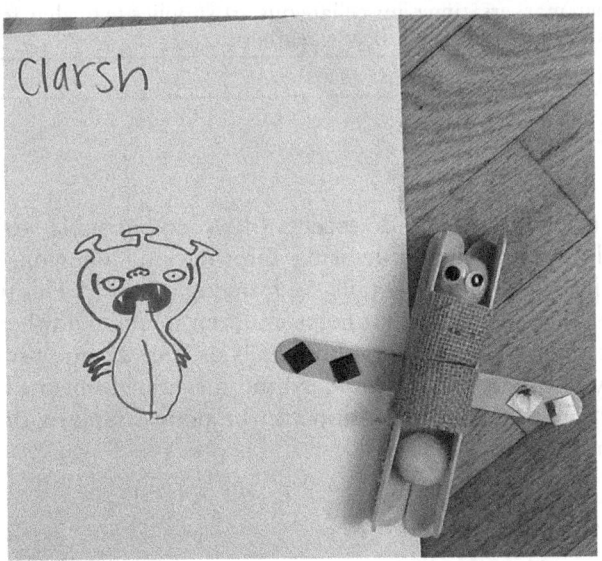

Figure 13.2 Clarsh example.

Sarah Moran

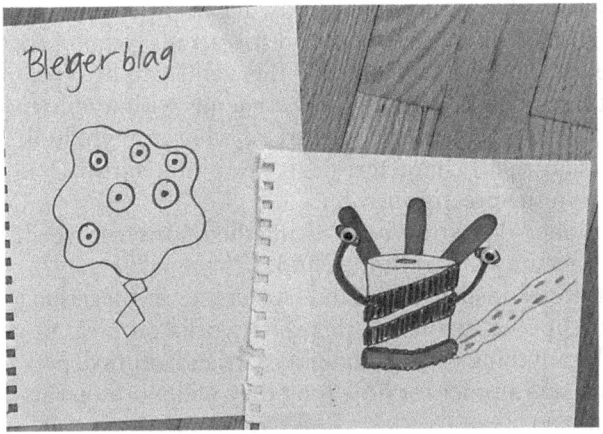

Figure 13.3 Blegerblag example.

Sarah Moran

7) This begins a discussion on how our brains are only able to create something we have an image of in our minds. The practitioner provides the example of making a peanut butter and jelly sandwich (PB & J) to demonstrate executive functioning. We only know how to make a PB & J because we have seen it made before and can follow the steps to get back to the final image in our minds. In this game, only the creator of a made-up word knows what it means, therefore there is no mind map on how to get there.

8) There are no wrong answers in this intervention. It may be valuable to share the reasons the child made the choices they made, such as the word sounds like this texture, or reminds me of a certain object. It is common for those who know each other well to have similar traits in their creations. This speaks to their level of connection and understanding of each other, and a sense of being seen.

Rationale

The goal of this play intervention is to highlight the creativity and strengths of all brains, as well as to educate the child on the process of executive functioning. It is typical to feel some anxiety when you are not sure of the plan or whether you are doing the exercise correctly, and this is comparable to the way we feel when asked to do something that our brains have no mind map for. This play intervention can be easily taught to parents and the parent and child can play the game at home, fostering connection. This play intervention could be used with a family or group therapy session, where one word is selected, and multiple people work to create the same nonsense word.

Greatness Cards

Therapy Needs: Strengths development, self-worth
Level: Child, adolescent
Materials: Deck of Greatness Cards developed by Tammi Van Hollander
Modality: Individual

Introduction

This play intervention utilizes Greatness Cards created by Tammi Van Hollander, which consist of several cards with strengths listed on them. The cards and specific game play are implemented to help the child identify their strengths. Tammi Van Hollander also created Greatness Sticks, which can be used instead of the cards.

Instructions

1) The practitioner shows the child the deck of Greatness Cards.
2) The practitioner explains that the child is going to go through the cards and make two piles. One pile is strengths they believe they have, and one is strengths they believe they do not have.
3) Once the piles are complete, the child is instructed to go through the strength pile and narrow it to ten cards they believe are their biggest strengths.
4) Once the ten are selected, the child is asked to go through the ten and select their top five. Once they have done this the child selects their top strength.
5) The practitioner and child talk about their top ten strengths and how they manifest in their life. They also discuss their number one strength and how much that strength is activated in their life.
6) The practitioner and child then look at the pile of strengths that they do not believe they have and see if there is one they would like to have as a strength in their life. If the child chooses one, the practitioner and child discuss how this could become a strength for the child.
7) The practitioner can take a picture of the child's top ten strengths and send it to the child to keep as a reminder.

Rationale

Neurodivergent children and adolescents possess strengths but often the strengths are not recognized or valued. This play intervention provides the opportunity for children to think about this concept and identify their top strengths. The strengths can be reinforced by the practitioner throughout therapy.

Look At My Strengths

Therapy Needs: Strengths development, self-worth, identity
Level: Child, adolescent
Materials: Construction paper, scissors, tape, marker
Modality: Individual, group

Introduction

Regardless of other therapy needs, it is important to help neurodivergent children and adolescents recognize and value their strengths. This intervention creates a strong visual which helps the child process and remember their strengths. It also assists the practitioner in better understanding the child's strengths and using these strengths to help address additional therapy needs.

Instructions

1) The practitioner explains to the child that they will be helping the child understand their strengths.

2) The practitioner provides the child with construction paper (different colors), scissors, a marker, and tape. The child is instructed to think about their strengths and cut out a piece of construction paper for each strength. Each piece of construction paper is a different strength, and the child should write the strength on the piece of construction paper. The child may not understand the concept of strengths and the practitioner may want to use different language such as, 'What do you like to do?', 'What do you think you are good at?', 'Where do you feel you have success?' Strengths can be many different things and the strengths the child indicates should not be minimized. Further, the practitioner can help suggest strengths they see in the child.

3) Once the child has completed all the strengths, they will tape each strength on themselves (arms, chest, etc.).

4) Once all the strengths have been taped on, the practitioner and child will look in a mirror and talk about each strength.

5) After the strengths have been discussed, the practitioner will take a picture of the child wearing all their strengths and send the picture to the child to keep and reference.

Rationale

Often neurodivergent children and adolescents receive feedback about what is 'wrong with them' and their 'problems'. There is little attention given to their strengths. This play intervention is designed to help children and adolescents recognize their strengths and improve their self-worth. Further, the practitioner can benefit from better understanding the child's strengths and utilizing these strengths to address other therapy goals.

Strengths Plate

Therapy Needs: Strengths development, self-worth, connection, and relationship development
Level: Child, adolescent
Materials: White paper plates, pen
Modality: Individual, group

Introduction

Strengths Plate is designed to help children and adolescents identify their strengths and understand that all people have strengths and things that are not their strengths. The practitioner completes this intervention with the child and provides some self-disclosure. The practitioner should consider their disclosures regarding how it best helps the child complete and understand the intervention.

Instructions

1) The practitioner tells the child they will be using a white paper plate to help identify strengths.
2) The practitioner and child try to think of as many strengths as they can and write them down on the side of the white paper plate. Any strength that either person can think of can be written on the plate.
3) Once this has been completed, the child's name is written at the top of the paper plate in the middle, and the partitioner's name is written at the top on the other side from the strengths.
4) Under the child's name, the child will put a check mark corresponding with any strength that was written down that they believe they have. Once the child is finished, the practitioner will do the same under their name.
5) The practitioner and child will then look at their check marks and compare – noting the strengths they share and noting differences.
6) The practitioner will want to point out that people have different strengths. They will also want to point out that people do not have strengths in everything, and it is okay to not have strengths in every area.
7) The child can keep the strengths plate and take it home as a reminder of their strengths.

Rationale

This play intervention helps children better understand their strengths and realize that everyone has different strengths, and it is okay to not have strengths in every area. The child can be encouraged to remember their strengths and understand that, although there may be some things they are not 'good at', they still have plenty of strengths.

Some Brains

Therapy Needs: Strengths development, identity, self-worth
Level: Child
Materials: The book *Some Brains: A Book About Neurodiversity* by Nelly Thomas, paper, markers or crayons
Modality: Individual

Introduction

This play intervention utilizes the children's picture book *Some Brains: A Book About Neurodiversity* by Nelly Thomas. Bibliotherapy is integrated with play therapy to help children recognize and appreciate strengths in the different ways their brain operates.

Instructions

1) The practitioner introduces the book *Some Brains* by Nelly Thomas and the practitioner and child read the book. The practitioner may want to read sections of the book or certain pages. The practitioner should decide this prior to implementing the intentions. Also, the book can be read by the practitioner, by the child, or they can take turns reading different pages.
2) Once the book has been read, the practitioner can ask the child what they thought about the book and what they thought was the message of the book.
3) After processing, the practitioner gives the child a piece of paper and some markers or crayons. The child is asked to draw a brain on the piece of paper.
4) This brain represents their brain. Once they have it drawn, they are instructed to write in the brain different things about their brain and anything they appreciate about their brain.
5) Once the child has finished, the practitioner asks them to share about their brain. The practitioner and child should process that their brain is okay and celebrate the things they appreciate.

Rationale

This play intervention is designed to help children better understand themselves, especially how their brain works. The purpose is to help children value and appreciate their brain and counter any negative messages that their brain differences are bad. The book reading and subsequent play intervention help reinforce these concepts. The practitioner may want to share the book with parents to purchase and read at home with their child.

Me and My Strengths

Therapy Needs: Strengths development, self-worth	
Level: Child, adolescent	
Materials: Paper, markers	
Modality: Individual, group, family	

Introduction

Neurodivergent children and adolescents may have never been introduced to the concept of strengths and do not understand that they have strengths. This is an expressive (drawing and coloring) play intervention that helps children identify strengths. Affirming note: Remember that the child's play preferences should be considered with implementing interventions. Some children may have a play preference for expressive creation interventions.

Instructions

1) The practitioner gives the child a piece of paper and markers or crayons.
2) The practitioner explains that they are going to work on identifying strengths
3) The practitioner asks the child to draw an outline of a person on their paper, covering most of the paper.
4) The practitioner asks the child to draw their own face and hair on the person.
5) For the rest of the person, the child is instructed to think about different strengths they have (the practitioner can help identify strengths), give each strength a color, and color it in their person somewhere.
6) The child can have as many strengths as they can think of, and they can indicate any type of strength.
7) Once the person is completed, the practitioner asks the child to share their strengths person, what strength goes with each color, and why they believe they have this strength.
8) The practitioner will want to encourage the child about their strengths and have the child take their strengths person home to keep and reference.

Rationale

Helping neurodivergent children to recognize and appreciate their strengths can be an ongoing progress. This play intervention provides the opportunity for children to identify and talk about their strengths and keep the person they created as a reminder of their strengths. Remembering and appreciating strengths will likely be an ongoing theme and interventions such as My Strengths Person can be revisited and completed in different sessions.

LEGO® Strengths

Therapy Needs: Strengths development	
Level: Child, adolescent	
Materials: Various LEGO® bricks	
Modality: Individual, group	

Introduction

Many neurodivergent children and adolescents have play preferences in constructive play, specifically in playing and building with LEGO® bricks. This play intervention uses LEGO® bricks to help children identify their strengths.

Instructions

1) The practitioner provides several LEGO® bricks that the child can use for the intervention.
2) The practitioner explains that they are each going to build something using the bricks. The theme of the build is a strength. The practitioner and child must think about a strength they have and represent it through a LEGO® build. The build can be something real or abstract. The strength can be represented in the construction design, color, or anything else related to the build.
3) Once the builds are complete, the practitioner will go first and share/explain their build – what it is and what strength it represents. The child will then share their build.
4) The practitioner and child can then make another build representing another strength. They can continue this play intervention until the child is no longer interested.

Rationale

LEGO® brick play can be a strong play preference for many neurodivergent children. This intervention utilizes brick building/creation to help children recognize their strengths. The child can create many builds for many strengths. They can be encouraged to create builds at home to represent their strengths and keep those builds in their room to remind them of their strengths.

Show and Tell (telehealth)

Therapy Needs: Strengths development, connection, and relationship development	
Level: Child, adolescent	
Materials: None	
Modality: Individual, family	

Introduction

This play intervention is best implemented through telehealth sessions. It can be done early in sessions to help both the child and therapist identify the child's strengths. It can also serve as an assessment intervention, allowing the practitioner to better know and understand the child.

Instructions

1) The practitioner explains to the child that when they say 'Go!', both the practitioner and child are going to leave the screen and go into their environment and find something that reminds them of a strength they have, something they do well, something they are proud of, etc.
2) Once both are back on their screen, the practitioner will go first and share what they found and talk about how it relates to the instruction. The child will go next and share the same.
3) This can be repeated with a new instruction. The practitioners and child can continue to play the intervention until the child is no longer interested.

Rationale

This play intervention helps the child identify strengths. It also helps the practitioner and child develop their relationship and the practitioner to learn more about the child. The home setting for the child often provides many opportunities for the Show and Tell intervention. It can be revisited in multiple sessions.

Teach Me

Therapy Needs: Strengths development, connection, and relationship development, executive functioning
Level: Child, adolescent
Materials: None
Modality: Individual, family, group

Introduction

Neurodivergent children and adolescents are often not allowed to show or have their strengths recognized. This play intervention provides the opportunity for the child to take the lead, share their knowledge, and teach something to the practitioner.

Instructions

1) The practitioner explains they are going to do an activity where the child will be teaching something to the practitioner.
2) The practitioner explains that the child is the 'expert', and the practitioner needs to learn the information.
3) The practitioner and child decide on what the child will be teaching or explaining to the practitioner. This is typically something the child knows

a lot about, possibly one of their special interests. It could be how to play a favorite video game, how to set up a social media account, all about LEGO. It can be anything the child has an interest in and knowledge about.

4) The practitioner's job is to listen and learn from the child. The practitioner should make the statement, 'Teach me all about this'.
5) The practitioner should ask questions and be genuinely interested in learning from the child.
6) Once the child is finished, the practitioner should thank the child for sharing their knowledge and provide some feedback on what they learned.

Rationale

This play intervention provides the opportunity for the child to feel confident and empowered. The teaching-the-practitioner element allows the child to share a strength regarding something they know a lot about and can help others learn. The practitioner should stay encouraging with the child and point out how much the child knows about the subject, and how they were able to help the practitioner increase their knowledge.

Rate Yourself 1–10

Therapy Needs: Strengths development, identity, connection, and relationship development
Level: Child, adolescent
Materials: Boogie Board
Modality: Individual

Introduction

This intervention is designed to be fun and encouraging of the child's strengths and identity as a neurodivergent person. The intervention utilizes a Boogie Board drawing/writing device but the practitioner could implement this intervention with paper and pencil.

Instructions

1) The practitioner provides a Boogie Board for the child and one for themselves.
2) The practitioner explains they are going to take turns making statements and then each of them will write on their Boogie Board a number from one to ten indicating how good they are at the statement. One indicates not good at all and ten indicates very good.

3) The statements should be a variety of types such as playing video games (or specific video games), feeding pets, getting dressed, math, drawing, relaxing, being short, fixing my hair, playing, etc.
4) The practitioner and child should take turns naming several things to rate. When a rating is provided, the practitioner and child can talk about why they provided that rating.
5) The practitioner should point out when the child rates themselves high in something and point out that people can't be good at everything and that is okay.

Rationale

This play intervention gives the child the opportunity to showcase things they are good at and recognize they have multiple strengths. It also provides the opportunity for the practitioner and child to discuss neurodivergence and how each neurodivergent person has strengths. The intervention can be repeated in multiple sessions to help solidify the child's awareness of their strengths.

Neurodiversity Puzzle

Therapy Needs: Strengths development, identity, self-worth
Level: Child, adolescent
Materials: Blank puzzle
Modality: Individual, family, group

Introduction

It is rare that information comes to a neurodivergent child that celebrates them as a neurodivergent person. In this intervention, a blank puzzle is completed with things that highlight the child or adolescent as a unique and awesome neurodivergent person.

Instructions

1) The practitioner gives the child a small, blank puzzle (typical size would be six puzzle pieces).
2) The practitioner explains that the child is going to turn the puzzle over and on each puzzle piece, they are going to write something that is valuable about themselves as a neurodivergent child. This may be a way they learn, socialize, express feelings, like to play, have sensory preferences, do with their free time, a physical ability, etc. The practitioner can help the child write and help them think of ideas.
3) Once the child has written something in each puzzle piece, the puzzle is turned over and the child can decorate/create the puzzle any way they like.

4) Once they have finished the puzzle, the practitioner and child will take it apart and put it back together.
5) As each piece is put together, the practitioner and child will talk about what the child wrote on that puzzle piece.
6) The child can take the puzzle home and complete it with their family.

Rationale

Neurodivergent children and adolescents need to know they are valuable and possess strengths as a neurodivergent person. So much of their experience is on what others identify they do wrong. This play intervention is designed to empower them to see themselves in a positive manner and recognize their neurodivergence from a strengths-based view.

Find the Toys

Therapy Needs: Strengths development, connection, and relationship development
Level: Child, adolescent
Materials: A variety of different types of toys, a blindfold
Modality: Individual, family

Introduction

This play intervention helps children and adolescents experience success. Children are typically blindfolded and led around the playroom by the practitioner. These instructions can be modified if needed to better fit the child. The practitioner will need to verify with the child they are okay to blindfolded and okay if the practitioner physically guides them around the playroom.

Instructions

1) The practitioner explains that the child will be blindfolded, and the practitioner will be leading them around the play therapy room to find specific toys.
2) Once the child is blindfolded, the practitioner tells them there are five toys to find and gives them the names such as a puppet, a person miniature, a ball, a hat, and car. The goal is for the child to experience success so the toys should not be difficult.
3) The practitioner will lead the child to one of the toys, they must feel around for it and when they get it, they have to name the toy correctly from the five options. If correct, they are then led to the next toy.
4) This continues until all five toys are found.
5) The practitioner and child can play the game as many times as they like using new toys. They can also switch roles and the child can lead the therapist.

6) The practitioner should encourage the child as they find toys, and after they have completed the task, they should point out how well the child did with accomplishing the game.

Rationale

This play intervention is designed to give the child or adolescent the opportunity to feel success and accomplishment. It is developed in a seek and find game format but should be easy enough for the child to complete. This intervention can be taught to parents to compete as a play time at home with their child.

Feeling Expert

Therapy Needs: Strengths development, feeling identification
Level: Child, adolescent
Materials: Feelings face cards, a feelings list, or any other product identifying feelings.
Modality: Individual, group

Introduction

This play intervention help children identify feelings that they understand and/or experience often. It also presents feeling awareness from a strength perspective, helping children recognize that feeling identification and awareness can be a strength.

Instructions

1) The practitioner tells the child that they will be doing a feelings identification game to discover what feelings the child is an 'expert' about.
2) The practitioner will provide the child with feelings cards or a feelings list.
3) The practitioner asks the child to pick out any feelings they believe they experience and /or understand well. These cards are placed in a pile.
4) Once the child has finished, the practitioner and child look at the feelings the child chose and discuss why the child chose those and believes they understand them well.
5) The practitioner can point out the child has a strength in understanding these feelings, as a lot of people do not understand feelings. If the child identified a negative feeling, the practitioner could point out that understanding a negative feeling is also a strength and can be very valuable to a person.
6) The practitioner can take a picture of the feeling strengths the child identified and send the picture to the child to keep at home.

Rationale

This play intervention simultaneously works on strengths awareness and feeling identification. It helps the child understand that feeling identification and awareness is a strength. Practitioners will need to be age appropriate when implementing this intervention (younger children may not be able to identify feelings) and observe for possible alexithymia issues.

14 Identity (Self-Worth) Interventions

Sketch, Sculpt, Print, and Paint (STEMpathic interventions)

(Contributed by Tony Vallance, Clinical Play Therapist)

Therapy Needs: Anxiety reduction, self-worth, empowerment, communication skills, empathic response skill building
Level: Child, adolescent
Materials: Pen and paper, playdough, 3D printer and acrylic paints/brushes, laptop/desktop computer with mouse.
Modality: Individual

Introduction

This externalization-based intervention involves the child initially reflecting on something that is a challenge or frustration for them (or someone they know – for some individuals it is easier to engage with this sort of intervention if they are creating solutions for others, then next time they can be scaffolded into creating solutions for their own challenges or solutions). Once the issue has been identified, they will sketch a device, gadget or object that can help to minimize or solve that problem. If appropriate as a sensory modality, the child can sculpt the design using playdough. Using free digital design software Tinkercad (www.tinkercad.com), the child is supported to create a digital representation of their design to be exported to the 3D printer. Once printed, they begin the process of painting the design. When completed, they process with the practitioner the features and benefits of the design they have created and are encouraged to talk about the product to both the practitioner and the parents. This play intervention builds on a project-based learning STEM (science, technology, engineering and mathematics) approach but is client-centered and designed to build skills and confidence in self-worth, empathic problem solving, creativity, 2D and 3D design, fine motor skills (painting the model), and communication (sharing about the model and how it will help them and/or others).

DOI: 10.4324/9781003398691-14

Instructions

1) The child is instructed to think about a particular frustration, challenge, or threat that they (or others) have to deal with.
2) They are then asked to sketch a gadget or device that can minimize or eliminate the identified issue.
3) Then they use playdough to sculpt a 3D representation of that device. Using free digital design software Tinkercad (www.tinkercad.com), they are supported to create a digital representation of their design to be exported to the 3D printer.
4) Then using acrylic paints, they are instructed to paint their creation (putting painted models on air purifiers is a good way to quickly dry them). With sculpting and painting, the practitioner can assist the child if needed.
5) Often a lot of organic sharing occurs while focusing on sculpting and painting.
6) Once completed, the child is encouraged to communicate about how their device solves a problem or helps with an issue. They may do so in front of the practitioner and their parents (if deemed appropriate)
7) The child can take their device home for display.

Rationale

Taking a solution-focused approach to child-identified issues can be extremely empowering. Particularly as they end up with a take-home device that they have sketched, sculpted, 3D designed, 3D printed, and painted. It also takes the child through contemporary, project-based learning steps most used in education with STEM/STEAM (science, technology, engineering, art, and mathematics) approaches that are a foundry for contemporary skills growth, such as creativity, design thinking, empathic problem solving, and communication. Often sharing occurs when the senses and concentration are engaged elsewhere such as with sketching, sculpting, and painting.

Terrific Tones

(Contributed by Tony Vallance, Clinical Play Therapist)

Therapy Needs: Anxiety reduction, self-worth, empowerment, executive function, feeling identification, communication
Level: Child, adolescent
Materials: Tongue drum (pentatonic), two mallets (one for the child, one for the practitioner)
Modality: Individual

Introduction

This play intervention serves as a good connection, transition, and introduction to a session. It involves using a tongue drum and creating the tones of your week, and then transitioning into a call and response memory game.

Instructions

1) The child is instructed to reflect on how their week has gone, the highlights and lowlights and then play the rhythm, intensity, and tones that match feelings about those events.
2) It should be around a 30-second to one-minute piece that the child plays.
3) The practitioner attempts to translate certain feelings experienced by the child based on what they heard and check in to see if they got it correct.
4) Initially, the practitioner may share the sound of their week to help model the intervention. This also enables the child to reflect on the sharing of the practitioner (empathic reasoning/perspective).
5) The pair decide collaboratively that the leader for the call and response part of this intervention plays either one, two or three notes at a time on the tongue drum (good for power and control dynamics). The follower must then repeat the notes back using their mallet.
6) The leader then plays the first notes and adds the same number on top, thus increasing the complexity (sometimes adding one note at a time is a good starting place for this activity).
7) The follower repeats and so on until they can't quite get the sequence. They switch places and reflect on the challenges of focusing, leading, and following.

Rationale

This play intervention uses the instrument of the tongue drum to assist in emotional expression, reflective practice, and empathic responding. The tongue drum is an instrument that has a low accessibility bar so only basic fine motor skills are required to strike it correctly. Changing roles between leader and follower unpacks understanding about power and control dynamics often seen with high anxiety and can be a helpful practice for some neurodivergent children.

Character Cards Evolution

(Contributed by Monica Fyfe, Registered Play Therapist Supervisor)

Therapy Needs: Self-worth
Level: Child, adolescent
Materials: Art supplies such as paper, color pencils, sharpies, Pokémon books/images/cards
Modality: Individual, family, group

Introduction

The concept of knowing one's own values in life is an integral part of the Acceptance and Commitment Therapy (ACT) model of psychology. Dixon and Paliliunas (2018) shared that 'values are not goals or objectives, rather they are the intangible ways you want to feel in this life, to make your life as important and meaningful as it can be' (p. 36). They also help us make decisions about the future. The focus of values work is to live one's life in a direction towards one's personal values, versus away from one's personal values. They are typically 'larger, later rewards' and not 'smaller, sooner' ones.

Some common examples of values may be Spirituality, Bravery, Risks, Creativity, Fun, Relaxation, Hard Work, Learning and Curiosity, Exploring, Adventure, Athletics and Exercise, Friends, Family, Helping Others and more.

This intervention adapts Acceptance and Commitment Therapy (ACT) for Play Therapy, by using age-appropriate language, choice, and experiential interventions for children and adolescents. ACT has also been used to support neurodivergent youth based on its integrative foundations of relational frame theory, functional and contextual behavior analysis, and mindfulness practices. A few important notes for this specific intervention for clinician to highlight within this directive play therapy intervention, are: *One's values help define your identity and who you are as an individual. Values commonly change over the lifespan. And one's values can be different than the values of family members.*

Instructions

1) The practitioner shares examples of age-appropriate characters that 'evolve' in form such as Pokémon (e.g., cards, toys, books, images, short videos may be used).
2) The practitioner and child pick a character card model that is motivating and interesting to the client. For example: Pichu evolves into → Pikachu by leveling up with a happiness value of 220. Pikachu can evolve into → Raichu when holding a Thunderstone upon leveling up. Those values shown may include Happiness, Bravery, Risks, Adventure.
3) The practitioner then passes out a blank page or provides choices of simple printable Character Card templates (there are many templates online, see references below).
4) The practitioner assists the child in brainstorming their values, health, strengths, weaknesses, powers, and more. This is an important time to highlight and affirm the child's strengths.
5) The practitioner encourages the child to create their own visual Character Idea and Character Name (while validating and enlarging the meaning of their self-as context identity choices).

6) The practitioner asks the child to decorate their own card. The practitioner can decorate their own card alongside the child to normalize and generalize the process and to note differences in others.
7) The practitioner and child can consent and choose to make copies (big or small), and laminate the images created by the child and practitioner.
8) The practitioner and the child can use these cards over time to play typical card games, to include all family members, similar to a genogram, and as an inspiring visual stored in all settings as a reminder of identity and selected values related to the child's daily choices.
9) After the intervention, the practitioner can choose to process the experience and to reflect on creating new cards in future sessions that show 'Transformation' and 'Evolutions' of the child over time, for added flexibility of one's changing identity.
10) In their Module 11 AIM interventions entitled 'Transformations,' Dixon and Paliliunas (2018) offer discussion prompts with child that may include:
    a. 'Do you think the values you have today will be the same for the rest of your life?
    b. 'Do you think they may change or evolve as you get older?'
    c. 'How have the things you cared about when you were five years old changed? How have they remained the same?'

Rationale

This play intervention helps children and adolescents understand values and what values they personally hold meaningful in their lives. It also helps children and adolescents to understand the difference between long-term deeper values vs short-term goals or rewards. It affirms their strengths and builds their self-worth. It also normalizes the concept that everyone has a different identity based on one's own choices. Lastly, it helps children and adolescents who may struggle with change, that their identity can mature and change over time, based on flexibility in their values and strengths. This intervention can be fun and effective in individual sessions, family therapy, and in groups. Children will gain the most benefit from this intervention if they revisit it periodically and update their character cards as they evolve in their psychological flexibility over time.

References

Dixon, M. & Paliliunas, D. (2018). AIM: Accept, Identify, Move. A Behavior Analytic Curriculum for Social-Emotional Development in Children. Shawnee Scientific Press.
Character Trading Card worksheet (n.d.): https://www.education.com/worksheet/article/character-trading-card/
Pokémon Card creator (n.d.): https://www.pokecard.net/

Self-Worth Conversation

Therapy Needs: Self-worth	
Level: Child, adolescent	
Materials: None	
Modality: Individual	

Introduction

Neurodivergent children often struggle with negative self-worth. Over time, their sense of self can become negative from many non-affirming experiences. This play intervention utilizes a conversation game to help the child strengthen their positive self-worth and dispel negative cognitions related to self.

Instructions

1) The practitioner gives instruction to the child that they are going to practice being in a conversation about themselves.
2) The practitioner gives the following instruction for how the conversation is going to flow back and forth: The practitioner is going to say something about themselves that they have thought or felt that was negative. The child is then going to say something they have thought or felt about themselves that was negative. These can also be written down on paper or in a conversation bubble sheet.
3) The practitioner will then say, 'I don't want to think or feel that about myself, I want to think about _____.' This will be competed with a strength, a positive cognition, something the practitioner likes about themselves. Then the child goes and says the same thing.
4) This process is completed several times, identifying negative cognitions and positives/strengths.
5) The practitioner should take advantage to reflect and discuss dispelling the negative cognitions and focusing on the strengths.
6) Play continues until the practitioner and child have covered several items or they are no longer interested in playing.

Rationale

Self-worth conversation helps children and adolescents work on improving their self-worth and dispelling negative cognitions about self. This play intervention should be practiced many times; in future sessions, the more a child can participate in this intervention, the more they can improve their self-worth. It is likely the child may not do well in the beginning and the practitioner may have to stop the intervention several times and give prompts to help the child identify positive cognitions and strengths. A positive cognitions and/or strengths list may be helpful for this intervention. Parents can be taught how to do this intervention at home with the expectation to practice with their child.

I Can Do That Game

Therapy Needs: Self-worth, regulation needs
Level: Child, adolescent
Materials: Index cards, pen, various toys
Modality: Individual, family, groups

Introduction

I Can Do That Game gives the practitioner and the child the opportunity to design a whole-brain movement intervention that is individualized to the child and creates a fun approach for the child to experience accomplishment and address regulation needs. This intervention can be especially helpful for children who prefer movement-based play.

Instructions

1) The practitioner divides index cards into three piles with about five to ten index cards in each pile.
2) The first set of index cards are action cards, the second set are object cards, and the third set are body part cards.
3) The practitioner and child write an action on each action card, such as jump three times, crawl on the floor, hop around the room, etc.
4) The practitioner and child write on each object card an object, such as with a ball, with a stuffed animal, with a toy car, etc.
5) The practitioner and child write different body parts on the body part cards, for example, under your chin, on your head, on your back, between your knees, etc.
6) Once the cards are complete, the practitioner and child play the game.
7) The child draws an action card first, then an object card, and last a body part card. The cards are put together and read something like this: (action) jump three times, (object) with a ball, (body part) on your head. The child then must complete the combination.
8) The practitioner should periodically reflect on the accomplishment of the child as they complete cards. The child and practitioner continue with the game until all the cards have been used.

Rationale

I Can Do That helps children and adolescents experience accomplishment to help improve their self-worth. The movement components (experienced by activating their whole brain) of the game can also help with regulation and sensory needs. This play intervention can be played repeatedly with new cards being made. The cards can be shuffled and played again with new combinations. Sample I Can Do That cards are available in the Appendix.

Good Me Mobile

Therapy Needs: Identity, self-worth, strengths
Level: Child, adolescent
Materials: Hanger, string, construction paper, markers
Modality: Individual

Introduction

Neurodivergent children and adolescents often struggle with understanding and valuing their neurodivergent identity. Creating a strong visual aid that helps them conceptualize their identity can be very empowering. Good Me Mobile is designed to create a strong visual aid that helps children remember their strengths, appreciate their differences, and feel positive about themselves.

Instructions

1) The practitioner and child cut out five pieces of different colored construction paper. Each piece gets one of the four categories written on it.
2) The child can choose which category goes with which color of paper.
3) The categories are Strengths, It's Okay To Be Different, What I Like, and Celebrate.
4) The practitioner and child glue or tape each of the four pieces of construction paper across a clothes hanger.
5) The practitioner and child then cut five pieces of string, each about a foot long, and tie them onto the hanger with one piece of string corresponding to each color/category.
6) The child and practitioner then cut out three pieces of construction paper for each of the five categories, so each category will have three more pieces of the same color cut out.
7) The child and practitioner will brainstorm things the child thinks, believes, or should consider for each category, such as what are the child's strengths, in what ways is the child different and that is okay, what the child likes about themselves, and what that child wants to celebrate about themselves.
8) The child and practitioner will write down responses and glue or tape them on the string underneath the corresponding category.
9) Once all four categories have been finished, the practitioner and child can read through each category and response and talk about the wonderful self of the child.

10) The practitioner may want to pair this intervention with a picture book (such as *Some Brains* by Nelly Thomas) or other resource that describes being neurodivergent in a positive manner.
11) The child takes the mobile home and keeps it in their room as a visual reminder.

Rationale

This play intervention helps children and adolescents understand and value themselves, especially as a neurodivergent person. It also helps create a positive sense of self and recognizes strengths. The mobile serves as a strong visual aid that the child can keep to remind them of their awesome selves.

My Olympics

Therapy Needs: Self-worth, executive functioning needs
Level: Child, adolescent
Materials: Various toys
Modality: Individual

Introduction

Neurodivergent children and adolescents may need help with executive functioning issues such as staying calm and maintaining focus and concentration in situations that move quickly. They also may need opportunities to increase their self-worth. This intervention provides a fun and engaging way for children and adolescents to work on these therapy needs.

Instructions

1) The practitioner and child set up several games to complete in the playroom. They should be simple games such as make three baskets in the basketball goal, draw a picture, punch the bop bag three times, hop across the sensory tiles, etc.
2) A series of games to complete is established by the practitioner and explained to the child.
3) The child must complete the games within a certain amount of time.
4) The practitioner discusses with the child that they will need to work on staying focused to complete all the games.
5) When the child is ready, the practitioner will say 'Go!' and the child will try to complete all the games. The practitioner will be timing the child.
6) Once the child completes all the games, the practitioner will tell them their time and ask them if they want to try again and see if they can get a faster time.

7) The practitioner and child can play as long as they want and create new games to complete. Once the child is finished, the practitioner and child make a special award ribbon for the child.

Rationale

This play intervention is designed to help children feel accomplished (improve their self-worth) and address executive functioning needs. The practitioner will want to make sure that the materials are available to complete several games. Table 14.1 lists several example games. Typically, around five to six games per session is an appropriate amount. Practitioners will want to challenge the child so they can work on staying focused and regulating this system. The practitioner will also want to process with the child how it felt to accomplish all the games. There should be time in the session to celebrate the child accomplishing the games and creating an award ribbon for the child.

Table 14.1 My Olympics Ideas

Make three baskets in a row
Solve a puzzle
Do a hoola hoop three times
Keep a balloon in the air for one minute
Complete a ring toss
Build something with blocks in 30 seconds
Hammer a nail into the wood
Find something buried in the sand tray
Walk across the playroom balancing a ball on your head
Draw a picture of you and your family
Solve a word scramble
Shoot targets with the nerf gun
Joust with the swimming pool noodles
Color a picture
Make something out of playdough
Run in place for one minute
Walk backwards around the room five times
Do not move for 20 seconds
Name 10 emotions in 30 seconds

Source: Grant, R. J. (2023)

My Way To Play

Therapy Needs: Self-worth	
Level: Child, adolescent	
Materials: Various toys	
Modality: Individual	

Introduction

Autistic and other neurodivergent children and adolescents typically have play preferences, ways they like to play that are meaningful to them. They may find that others devalue their play preferences and try to make them play in ways they deem appropriate. This intervention is designed to empower the neurodivergent child to understand there is not one 'right' way to play, to freely engage in play the way they like, and to feel positive about their play preferences.

Instructions

1) The practitioner instructs the child that they are going to have a play time.
2) The practitioner explains the concept of play preferences and that there is no one or right way to play.
3) The practitioner explains to the child they get to choose what they play and how they play and can play in any way they like. The practitioner will ask the child if they know how they like to play and what their interests are.
4) The practitioner explains that the child will lead out in their play preference and the practitioner will participate as the child wants.
5) As the play is happening, the practitioner should periodically reflect that there is no 'right' way to play and validate the child's play preferences. The practitioner may also disclose their own play preferences or preferences they have seen from others.
6) Play will likely continue until the session is finished.

Rationale

This play intervention helps children appreciate and feel positive about the way they like to play. It is designed to help improve the child's self-worth and counter any negative experiences they have had with others judging their play and interests as wrong, bad, or weird.

Interview Me

Therapy Needs: Identity, self-worth, social navigation	
Level: Child, adolescent	
Materials: Paper, pencil	
Modality: Individual, family, group	

Introduction

This intervention helps children and adolescents work on identity awareness, self-worth, and social navigation related to asking other people questions, and learning about others. It is also an interactive intervention between the practitioner and child, which helps support relationship development.

Instructions

1) The child is instructed that they and the practitioner are going to interview each other.
2) The child is given a piece of paper and a pencil and asked to come up with seven questions to ask the practitioner. The practitioner will do the same for their interview of the child.
3) The practitioner's questions for the child should help support the child's identity and feeling positive about themselves. They should be open-ended questions, avoiding yes or no response questions. Some sample questions include: What is your favorite thing in this playroom? What do you like to do in your free time? What do you know you do well? What are three positive thing you have heard other people say about you? What do you like best about yourself today? What should be celebrated about you?
4) If the child is struggling to think of questions for the practitioner, then the practitioner can offer some example questions, such as: What is your favorite thing to do? Tell me about your family. Do you have a favorite vacation?
5) Once the practitioner and child have written their questions, they will take turns asking each other the questions and recording the answers.
6) The practitioner and child can practice through several interviews if there is time.
7) The child can then be instructed to go home and interview someone in the same format, using the same guidelines, and bring the interview to the next session.

Rationale

This play intervention helps children and adolescents work on identity aware-ness and self-worth, as well as social navigation related to asking questions, listening, and staying focused in a conversation. The child may struggle with coming up with appropriate interview questions, recording the practitioner's responses, and with completing the interview. At any point, the practitioner can stop the intervention and help the child focus. The practitioner can also con-sider if the interview needs to be shorter, with fewer questions. It will likely take practice for the child to complete this intervention without some help from the practitioner. Parents should be made aware that the child may be completing an interview at home and assist their child in completing the intervention.

Quiet and Loud

Therapy Needs: Identity, self-worth, body awareness
Level: Child, adolescent
Materials: None
Modality: Individual, group

Introduction

Neurodivergent children often have a different way of navigating. Other peo-ple may not always appreciate the child's neurotype and the child may receive negative messages about themselves. This intervention uses body awareness to help children understand they are valuable and fine, no matter who they are, how they feel, and what they do.

Instructions

1) The practitioner tells the child that they are going to do some activities that help the child appreciate being themselves.
2) The practitioner first expresses that sometimes we may feel quiet and sometimes we may feel loud. We can feel however we feel, and this is okay. The practitioner demonstrates pressing their hands together in front of them and begins by saying this is our way of being quiet.
3) The practitioner and child practice saying things quietly and tip-toeing around the room. The practitioner explains that sometimes in some situ-ations we may feel like being quiet and this is okay.
4) The practitioner moves their hands all the away apart and until both arms are fully stretched out. The practitioner explains this is our way of being loud.
5) The practitioner and child practice saying things loudly and stomping around the room. The practitioner explains that sometimes, in some situ-ations, we may feel like being loud and this is okay.

6) The practitioner can follow up the activity by discussing times and situations where they have felt quiet or loud in their thoughts and body. The practitioner and child can also practice more examples of quiet and loud.

Rationale

This play intervention works on increasing awareness and acceptance of self. Body movement is utilized to better help the child connect to their understanding of their neurodivergent self. It is likely that this intervention will need to be played multiple times to help the child progress in self-worth, especially related to their neurodivergence. Parents can be taught to complete this intervention at home with their child.

Construction Paper Face

Therapy Needs: Identity awareness
Level: Child, adolescent
Materials: Construction paper, glue, scissors, pen
Modality: Individual, group

Introduction

This play intervention helps children recognize and connect with their identity as a neurodivergent person. With this intervention, children identify different parts of themselves through a strength, positive, and it is okay to different lens. The practitioner may also provide psychoeducation on what it means to be neurodivergent and emphasize empowerment in differences.

Instructions

1) The practitioner explains to the child that they will be making faces using construction paper.
2) The child chooses a piece of paper that will represent their face. They cut out a large circle to represent their head.
3) The child then puts a face on the paper using construction paper only. The child will cut out eyes, eyebrows, ears, nose, mouth, hair, etc. from construction paper. The child is instructed to make their face however they like.
4) Once the child has completed making the face, the practitioner shares with the child that they are going to write on the different parts of the face strengths and positive things about the child.
5) The practitioner can help the child identify strengths and positives. Each one is written on a facial feature or somewhere on the face.
6) The practitioner and child should discuss each strength and positive as they are written on the face. The practitioner should also affirm the child's neurodivergence and any neuro differences the child may possess.

Rationale

This play intervention is designed to help children understand and value their identity, improve their self-worth, and feel positive about their differences. The practitioner and child can create multiple construction faces with different parts of the child represented. The practitioner can teach this intervention to parents to complete at home with their child.

This is Me Mane

Therapy Needs: Identity, self-worth
Level: Child
Materials: White paper plates, markers, string, hole punch
Modality: Individual, group

Introduction

This is Me Mane provides neurodivergent children the opportunity to better recognize parts of themselves, especially strengths and positives. This is an expressive art intervention that incorporates a visual and tactile component, creating a more sensory. The practitioner can help the child with the construction elements if needed.

Instructions

1) The practitioner communicates to the child that they will be creating a mane (like a lion's mane) that the child will be able to wear around their face.
2) The practitioner and child cut out the center of a white paper plate. The center piece is thrown away and the rest of the paper plate ring is colored with different colors (only the underneath side of the plate ring is colored).
3) Each color represents a different strength or positive they child believes about themselves or feeling that the child experiences sometimes.
4) The strength/positive/feeling word for each color should be written on the inside of the paper plate ring corresponding to the color that represents that item.
5) Once the plate has been colored, a hole is punched on each side and string is used to tie in each hole and make an open mask that can be tied on the child's head.
6) The finished product will resemble a lion's mane look. Once the mane is on the child's head, the child should look in a mirror and go through each strength/positive/feeling (whatever was the focus) and discuss it further. Figure 14.1 provides an example of a completed This is Me Mane.

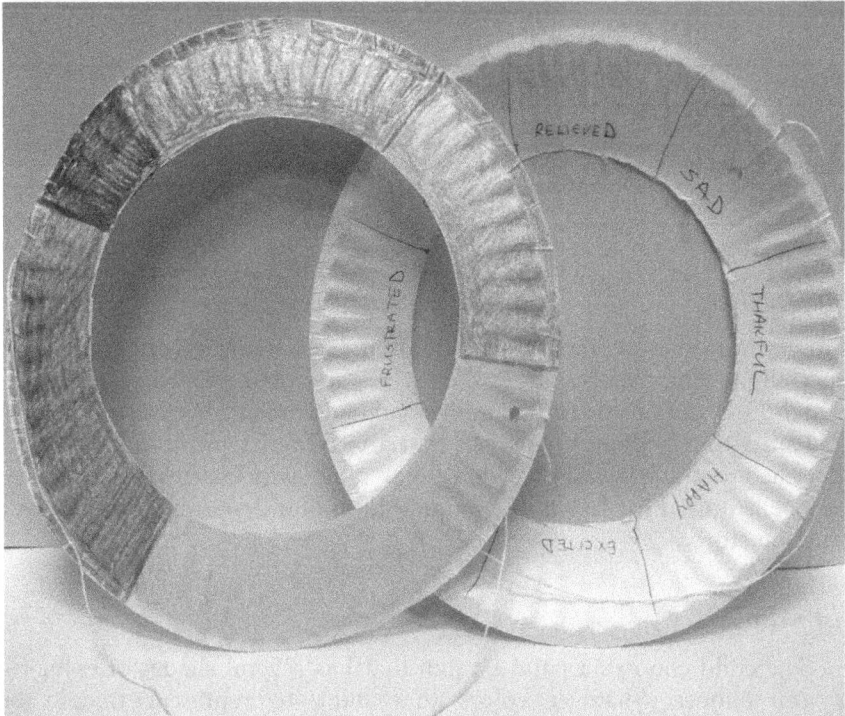

Figure 14.1 This is Me Mane.

Robert Jason Grant

7) The practitioner should empower the child with the identified strengths and positives and affirm the message that different is okay. If completing a feeling version, the practitioner should discuss with the child how the child has different feelings inside of them at different times and it is okay to experience different feelings and learn to identify them.

Rationale

This play intervention helps children work on improving their self-wroth, recognizing strengths, and identifying and understanding feelings. Completing this intervention periodically will help the child better understand their neurodivergence and improve their self-worth. Wearing the mane and discussing the items while looking in a mirror can help the child to connect with and take ownership of the process. These elements also provide a strong visual element to the intervention; the child can keep the mane and have it at home for reference.

Paint Swatch Pieces of Me

Therapy Needs: Identity, self-worth
Level: Child, adolescent
Materials: Paint swatches, pen
Modality: Individual, group

Introduction

Autistic and other neurodivergent children often struggle with their identity, especially feeling positive about themselves and their neurodivergence. Paint Swatch Pieces of Me provides children and adolescents with the opportunity to identify things about themselves that are strengths, positive, and that they like. The practitioner will provide several paint swatch strips. These can typically be acquired for free in the paint section of a department or home construction store.

Instructions

1)   The child chooses a paint swatch that has several shades of color (they can choose whatever colors they like), to represent things about themselves.
2)   The practitioner explains that they are going to write on each color of the paint swatch something the child thinks is a strength they have, something positive about themselves, or something they like about themselves.
3)   The child should think of as many things as they can (they can use multiple paint swatches if needed). The practitioner can also help the child identify positive things.
4)   Once the child has finished writing their ideas, the practitioner and child talk about each one and how it contributes an important piece to the child's identity.
5)   The practitioner can further the intervention by asking the child to rank the things identified, from the most important part of their identity to the least important. The practitioner and child can then discuss the child's rankings.
6)   The child should keep the paint swatch as a visual reminder of the important parts of their identity.

Rationale

Many neurodivergent children struggle with low self-worth and a negative view of their neurodivergence (often having internalized ableism). Paint Swatch Pieces of Me helps children and adolescents strengthen identity awareness as a neurodivergent person and feel positive about themselves and the components that make up who they area. Several paint swatches can be created to identify multiple positives and strengths about the child. Paint swatches can be acquired for free at various hardware and paint stores.

I am a Tree, We are a Family

Therapy Needs: Identity, self-worth, connection, attachment
Level: Child
Materials: None
Modality: Family, group

Introduction

I am a Tree, We are a Family is implemented in a family or group setting. This play intervention promotes understanding and appreciating yourself (uniqueness and differences), connecting with other people, and working together to accomplish a task. This intervention requires no props or materials but typically a minimum of three people are needed to complete the intervention.

Instructions

1) The practitioner explains to the family that they will be working together to create a short and fun skit that they will perform for the practitioner.
2) The practitioner should designate a stage area in the room where the skit will be performed.
3) The family must choose one person who will lead out the skit and be the tree. The tree goes first and moves to the stage area, makes a tree shape, and says, 'I am a Tree.'
4) The family must decide who will go second, third, and so on. Each person will be something different that naturally connects to a tree. Some examples might be grass, leaves, roots, a bird, a squirrel, a piece of fruit, an acorn, moss, etc.
5) For example, the second person to go might be a leaf. That person would go next and move to the stage area, physically connect (however they choose) to the 'tree' person and say, 'I am a leaf.'
6) Then the third person would go and so on. Once the last person has gone, then the family says in unison, 'We are a family.'
7) The family should be given as much time as they need to create the skit (although it will likely not take long). They will need to decide the order that each person will go and what each person will be. Once the family has finalized the skit, they will perform the skit in front of the practitioner. If the family would like, they can perform a second skit with each family member choosing different parts to perform.

8) The practitioner should celebrate their connection and working together, and each of their differences and how they all are valuable and connect.

Rationale

This play intervention helps children work on appreciating who they are (their differences), connection, and relationship development, especially in the areas of understanding what everyone brings is important, attuning to other people, and working as a group to accomplish a task. The practitioner should give the full instruction to the family before they begin and then allow them time to put together their skit. Once the skit has been performed, the practitioner should applaud and congratulate the family. The practitioner might suggest creating additional skits with each family member leading as the tree.

My Social Navigation Puzzle

Therapy Needs: Identity, social navigation needs and questions, self-awareness, empowerment
Level: Child, adolescent
Materials: Small blank puzzle (blank puzzles can be ordered from several places online including Amazon.com), markers, pencil
Modality: Individual, familygroup

Introduction

This intervention helps children express their thoughts, strengths, and questions related to their social navigation world. The puzzle element provides a visual, tactile, and engaging element to conceptualizing and sharing information. This intervention can be especially helpful for children who have a play preference in art and/or creative expression.

Instructions

1) The practitioner explains to the child that they will be creating a puzzle that helps the child express their thoughts about their social world.
2) Using a small blank puzzle (six pieces for younger children, six to nine pieces for adolescents), the child writes on the back of each puzzle piece a different social strength, question, or thought they have about navigating their social world. The practitioner may need to spend time talking about what is meant by social world – the child's navigation and experience with school, public places, friends, being around other people in person or online, etc. The practitioner may also need to explain strengths – what you think feels good, that you like, that you think you do well in these scenarios. The practitioner should also encourage the child to write

down anything they have a question about or wonder about. The child can write down any combination of these things as they relate to their social world.

3) On the front of the puzzle, the child can decorate the puzzle however they want. They can create a picture or color the puzzle randomly – it is their design.

4) Once the child is finished, the practitioner and child then take the puzzle apart and put it back together. Each time a piece is connected, the practitioner and child can talk about what the child wrote down on that piece – a strength, question, or thought. The practitioner and child can take the puzzle apart and put it back together, discussing the pieces multiple times.

5) As social navigation questions and thoughts are discussed, the practitioner will make sure to remain neurodiversity-affirming in their responses to the child. This can be a powerful opportunity to help the child feel positive about their neurodivergent identity and strengthen their self-worth. Navigating differently is not wrong, different is okay!

Rationale

Many neurodivergent children and adolescents are inundated with messages that their way of navigating is wrong, bad, a problem, etc. This often leads to unhealthy concepts like masking and lowering the child's self-worth. My social navigation puzzle can help children and adolescents recognize and affirm their social-related strengths and provide the opportunity to address questions and thoughts they have about their social world. Parents can be involved in this play intervention and complete the puzzle at home with their child. Parents and children can also create new puzzles. Affirming note: Practitioners will want to make sure parents understand neurodiversity-affirming practices before having parents implement interventions at home.

15 Advocacy Interventions

My Fantastic Brain

(Contributed by Robyn Rausch Registered Play Therapist Supervisor™)

Therapy Needs: Advocacy, self-worth, identity, executive function needs
Level: Child, adolescent
Materials: Choose an approach that fits developmental age and neurotype qualities and preferably emphasizes their natural cognitive strengths.
Option 1 – Words: Colorful writing utensils of different sizes and types (big/small, crayon, marker, pens, etc.), paper (8in. x 11in. or larger)
Option 2 – Creation: Boxes, manila folders, paper, colorful writing utensils of different sizes and types (big/small, crayon, marker, pens, etc.), large variety of stickers or magazine photos, various other art supplies as available (popsicle sticks, puff balls, glitter, etc.)
Option 3 – Toys: Fully stocked play therapy office and/or sand tray office, table, paper, or rug
Modality: Individual, family, group

Introduction

Neurodivergent children and adolescents often find themselves not meeting the 'standards' set by schools, adults, and peers. These standards are often based on neurotypical strengths and weaknesses, and may imply that the strengths of neurodivergent brains are less important or even problematic. This results in individuals who are unable to recognize their own strengths, much less value them. This activity can be completed in one session or can be spread across multiple sessions to allow deeper reflection and self-awareness growth. This play therapy intervention is set up with three options which allows the client and practitioner to choose the approach that best fits the client's developmental age and neurotype. Choosing the approach is the first step in the intervention as it asks the practitioner and child to work together to begin identifying the cognitive strengths that will make this activity most beneficial. The following qualities should be considered when choosing:

DOI: 10.4324/9781003398691-15

Option 1: Low movement, low sensory input, requires language, particularly fitting for those who are highly logical and informational in their thinking.

Option 2: Moderate movement, moderate to high sensory input, no language needed, messy and less controlled, particularly fitting for those who struggle with attention control and are highly resourceful and creative in their thinking.

Option 3: High movement, high sensory input, no language needed, concrete symbols, particularly fitting for those who are very intuitive and relational in their thinking.

Instructions

1) The practitioner introduces the activity by explaining that there are many types of brains in the world. Just like there are many breeds of puppies, like Chihuahuas or Golden Retrievers. Puppies in each breed are very much like one another, but not exactly the same. Brains also have many types like Autistic, Anxious, or Neurotypical. The funny thing is sometimes we only think about neurotypical brains, even though this group is not even that common. This activity is one that lets us focus on what is fantastic about your type of brain. But we have choices in how we want to complete the activity.

2) Support the client by identifying what materials they would like to use from the options above. Options are meant to give a starting place: feel free to combine or improvise more materials.

   a. Option 1: Have both materials ready in a comfortable workspace for writing and explain the paper is supposed to represent the child's brain.

   b. Option 2: Choose either a box, a folder, or a paper to represent the child's brain for the project. Have the rest of the materials readily available and in a workspace that can get messy.

   c. Option 3: Set out a paper, table, or rug that designates a specific space to represent the child's brain.

3) One at a time, name each characteristic of a neurotype listed below and explain what some different brains do. Then have the child identify what their brain does for this characteristic and use their materials to represent it (Option 1: write it on the 'child's brain'; Option 2: choose or make a symbol and attach it to the 'child's brain'; Option 3: choose a toy symbol to place on the 'child's brain').

4) Help the child identify how each characteristic is a strength. Ask questions together such as 'How does this help me figure things out'? 'How does this help me be or feel safe'? 'What kind of job relies on this skill'? 'What kind of extracurricular relies on this sport'? 'How does it help my friends and family that I have this skill'?

5) Ask the client to celebrate their amazing brain type and all these skills with you. For example, they may dance, decorate it, give it an award, etc. Table 15.1 provides an example of neurotype qualities, characteristics, and strengths.

Table 15.1 Examples of Neurotype Qualities, Characteristics, and Strengths

Neurotype Qualities	Example Characteristics	Description	Benefits
Zoom Lens	Detail focus	Sensory observation skills that record millions of details instantly and bring most into awareness rather than filtering by priority.	More resourcefulness, more creativity in using information or objects, better able to identify mistakes.
	Big picture focus	General sensory observation skills that misses details but can observe and make sense of enough to develop a clear storyline or understanding of the area or events.	Excellent at problem solving and conflict resolution, more goal orientation, and efficiency.
	Pattern focus	Sensory observation skills that hones in on patterns and discards isolated and presumed unnecessary details.	Excellent at sorting information and identifying predictable patterns. Excellent intuition.
	Relationship focus	Sensory observation skills that hones in on relationships such as cause and effect, bi-directional, mutually beneficial, and parasitic and discards presumed confounding variables.	Excellent at making predictions and assumptions. Easily recognizes the impact of changes on other people, events, or ideas.
Processing Speed	Slow	Information evaluation skills that prioritizes accuracy over urgency and is cautious, detailed, and inductive in nature.	Very thorough understanding of new ideas. Less likely to make careless mistakes. More likely to notice confounding variables.
	Medium	Information evaluation that balances the priorities of accuracy and urgency.	Balances understanding and clarity with the need for urgency resulting in highly efficient productivity.
	Fast	Information evaluation that prioritizes decision making and urgency over accuracy and is fast, rule based, and deductive in nature.	Quickly processes lots of information and draws a conclusion allowing for quick decisiveness. Usually excellent at adapting to new information.
	Variable	Information evaluation that has a gear shift allowing the individual to change speeds depending on the situation.	More control over how thorough and how quickly they process information. Better able to determine and adapt to situations here either urgent or accuracy is more important.

Thinking Palette	Black and White	Thinking that involves all or nothing; yes or no; right or wrong labeling; and decision making.	Strong sense of class and beliefs. Highly loyal, high integrity, high congruence.
	Grayscale	Thinking that involves a continuum of ideas and possibilities which can be easily adjusted flexibly to accommodate new information or different scenarios.	Easily makes small adjustments allowing them to find a precise solution to changing situations. Greater empathy and understanding for other people's ideas even when they contradict one's own beliefs.
	Crayon	Thinking that involves a selection of ideas and possibilities that are chosen individually and applied in specific scenarios but are more difficult to adjust in small ways.	More creative and resourceful than the other two. Able to understand the pros and cons of any idea, object, or event from many perspectives and see the potential uses and opportunities that lie ahead. More difficulty making decisions and committing to a path.
Train Tracks	Express Line	Direct logical thinking that has a termination point, and no natural follow up. At the end of the line, the thought or idea is set down and the individual moves on to something new.	Highly productive, Results driven, Fact based, and quick to respond and process new information.
	Switch Track	Thinking that has train switches that allow the individual to shift to nearby ideas and opportunities easily.	Excellent at creativity, exploration, and curiosity. Inventive and elaborate in their ideas.
	Circuit Track	Circular thinking that often has a home station where the topic periodically returns.	Grounded in core beliefs that create consistency and predictability. Easily remains goal focused and on task.

(Continued)

Table 15.1 (Continued)

Neurotype Qualities	Example Characteristics	Description	Benefits
Attention Control	Persistent	Attention that works like a strong magnet finding an interesting target and refusing to release without great effort.	Can often work in any environment. More reliable short term and working memory allowing for efficient productivity. Goal focused.
	Controlled	Attention that works like a switchboard where the individual can control when attention moves easily.	Requires the individual make choices about how to use attention efficiently and allows for greater flexibility with new ideas and information as well as more adaptability in transitions. Efficient productivity comes from the ability to reduce time spend on transitions and getting "back in the groove."
	Distractible	Attention that works like sand, blowing around in a seemingly chaotic manner when impacted by wind and settled and still only when left on itself.	High energy, creative, inventive, and resourceful. Collects interesting or novel ideas for use later. High interest in exploring and learning new things making them more development and growth focused on their work.
Adaptability	Water	Ideas that are easily shifted by simply changing the environment or context.	Consistency is traded for flexibility allowing the individual to work in many environments and with many other types of brains in efficient and positive ways. Allows for creativity and adaptability.
	Pool Noodle	Ideas that change and are flexible enough to fit different contexts most but retain a core purpose and value.	Retains core values and focus allowing integrity and goal focused decision making. Particularly productive with people who have similar brain types if they are also flexible to some degree. Difficulty working with pool ladders (see below). Highly resourceful and creative.

Pool Float	Ideas that have some flexibility when pressure is applied and consistent, but if too much flexibility is required the idea snaps and confusion and panic follow as the child tries to fix it.	Strong values and congruence. High integrity and goal focus. Ability to adjust to changes especially if given time to prepare or process the changes. Difficulty working with other brain types in collaborative projects, but excellent at parallel work with anyone.
Diving Board	Ideas that have moderate flexibility and significant strength due to heavy core values. Ideas will flex appropriately to certain situations, but simply refuse to go any further when straying far from the original. There is no confusion or panic, the individual simply will not listen, agree, or comply.	Integrity and loyalty are unmatched. Highly consistent and predictable making them easy to collaborate with if you agree with their core values and beliefs about the world. Easily works with floats, noodles, and water, but struggles to collaborate with ladders and other diving boards.
Pool Ladder	Ideas that have no flexibility and significant strength. The individual becomes oppositional to any pressure to adjust their ideas.	Highly productive and efficient within their skills and values. They work quickly and with few careless errors. Excellent at explaining, reasoning, and remembering details about their beliefs. Difficulty working with other people unless that are highly matched on values, beliefs, and goals.

(Continued)

Table 15.1 (Continued)

Neurotype Qualities	Example Characteristics	Description	Benefits
North Pole	Connection	Thoughts that focus on and prioritize relationships, people, and community. What will this mean to others and how will it affect them?	Excellent coworker or friend as they are highly responsive and empathetic. They trade decisiveness for precision and thoroughness. Fantastic at noticing cause and effect relationships if people are directly impacted.
	Capability	Thoughts that focus on and prioritize skill, achievement, and status. What will this give me and how can I use it?	Highly motivated and productive. Easily sets goals and is easily reinforced through praise and rewards causing them to build new habits easier than most. Highly interested in growth and learning.
	Counting	Thoughts that focus on and prioritize meaning, influence, impact, and legacy. What will this change in the world, and will it change anything?	Skilled at long term planning and big picture assessments. Wastes little energy or resources. Trades initiative and urgency for thoughtfulness and efficiency.
	Courage	Thoughts that focus on and prioritize strength, power, and weighing risks against benefits. How can I do this and limit the risks, and how can I overcome other problems using it?	Willing to take calculated risks when appropriate to further a goal. Decisive and driven to make progress. Resourceful and excellent at problem solving.

Source: Robyn Rausch

Rationale

Neurodivergent children and adolescents often feel like outsiders who cannot do things they 'should be able to do' according to ableist and neurotypical standards. While most of the world focuses on neurotypical strengths, this activity asks the child to focus on the strengths of their neurotype and symbolize them in a concrete way that can make a lasting impression on their mind. Seeing all their strengths covering a paper, craft, or table demonstrates clearly how 'full of superpowers' their brain is, and how many amazing skills they can do (the practitioner might even point out to them that some of their strengths are ones their neurotypical peers usually struggle with).

The language used in the description of 'brain types,' also called neurotypes, is intentionally chosen to reinforce the idea that brains come in many types and even within those types, everyone is unique. It seeks to erase neurotypical as the standard brain that all skills and behaviors should be compared to and replace it with the idea of brains that are more like a box of crayons where all the colors are perfect for one task or another.

The options of how to execute this activity are also intentionally chosen to begin the practical application of different brains by emphasizing that not all brains would like any one approach. The conversation begins with what their brain loves and is 'really good at.' The product itself becomes an example of their greatest skills at work.

Steppingstones Game

Therapy Needs: Advocacy, relationship development, social navigation
Level: Child, adolescent
Materials: Card stock, foam pieces, Sharpie, small prize
Modality: Individual, family, group

Introduction

Neurodivergent children and adolescents often encounter challenges navigating various environments that do not value their neurodivergence. In these environments, children may need to advocate for their preferences and needs (for others to be accepting of their neurotype processes). This intervention creates a game format that can be played repeatedly which focuses on helping children and adolescents gain advocacy knowledge and ability.

Instructions

1) The child cuts out six to eight pieces of foam in the shape of steppingstones.
2) The foam pieces are then glued on a piece of card stock in the formation of a path, with a designated beginning and end.

3) The practitioner and child then decide on a situation or environment the child is typically in that seems devaluing of the child (the practitioner may need to help with the selection of the environment).
4) The situation or environment is written somewhere on the card stock and the child can then decorate the rest of the card stock in any way they want; at the end of the last steppingstone, the child should write 'PRIZE!' Providing a prize at the end of the game is optional but can be a fun and celebratory piece for the child.
5) The final piece of construction is to write an advocacy idea for the targeted situation or environment on each steppingstone. The practitioner should provide the opportunity for the child to think of ideas, but the practitioner will likely need to share ideas, as most children will be learning how to advocate. Advocacy ideas will vary from child to child and environment to environment. Some general ideas to teach include body autonomy, sharing you are uncomfortable, or you do not like something, asking for help, telling someone you need something such as a break, a change, a sensory adjustment, etc.
6) The practitioner and child then play the steppingstones game. Keeping the situation or environment in mind, the child starts at the beginning stone and reads the advocacy idea. The practitioner and child then practice the idea in a role-play. Once it has been practiced, the child receives a chip, token, or penny.
7) The child then moves on to stone two and repeats the process until they get to the end. They can then turn in all their chips and receive a small prize.

Rationale

Steppingstones helps children and adolescents work on understanding what advocacy is and how they can advocate for themselves. This is an important empowering construct for neurodivergent children and adolescents as they will enter many environments where they will need to advocate. Situations and environments that are real and tend to be struggle situations for the child should be chosen for the game. Practitioners may want to consult with parents and include them in the game for a family play session. The practitioner should ask the child (and parents) to identify advocacy ideas, but the practitioner will likely be providing psychoeducation about advocacy and will need to share ways to advocate. The Autism Level Up program provides free resources with many accommodations and advocacy ideas. This is a resource that can be used in this game and shared with families.

Initiations

(Contributed by Monica Fyfe Registered Play Therapist Supervisor™)

Therapy Needs: Advocacy, connection, relationship developmental, social navigation
Level: Child

Materials: Preferred toys of the child based on their own unique interests and motivation
Modality: Individual, family

Introduction

This intervention is informed from JASPER principles (a specific model of therapy that focuses on joint attention, symbolic play, engagement, and regulation).. Engagement in all children has been described in the developmental model in Adamson et al. (2004). The highest state of engagement with others is called *joint engagement*. This is where children can connect and coordinate their interactions through play, joint attention, noticing people and objects, and importantly initiate their thoughts with others. Very young Autistic and other neurodivergent children often spend a lower amount of time during their social interactions in a joint engagement state (Adamson et al., 2004). Kasari et al. (2022) noted that 'in order to coordinate interactions and enter the highest states of engagement, the child must be able to initiate ideas of their own, not just follow the adult' (p. 20).

Neurodivergent children may not feel comfortable, accepted, or allowed to be themselves, and initiate/participate with others. In addition, the issue of consent for neurodivergent youth prior to therapy and during therapy is a significant area for practitioners to be consistently aware of. Historically, many neurodivergent clients have reported later in life as adults that they were not in assent with many interventions and therapies they participated in as a child. By collaborating on a goal of increased initiations, the practitioner and family can encourage greater and more natural opportunities to follow the child's own generated and shared ideas.

Instructions

1) This play intervention is non-directive. It most closely aligns with a child-centered play therapy approach that is informed by development, language, connection, engagement, and self-advocacy.
2) The practitioner should place toys in the child's play environment that are of high interest and motivation to their own unique and individualized interests. Many choices are helpful to keep engagement and interest high. However, practitioners may need to reduce distractions of too many play items, if observed as a competing factor in the environment by the child.
3) The practitioner should pay close attention to novel play actions, themes and signs of interest, and follow the child's lead.
4) Kasari et al. (2022) described four tips on how to indirectly support and expand the child's verbal or non-verbal *Initiations* and joint attention during sessions together. These included: introducing interesting toys or actions for play story expansions and combinations (such as from another play theme or category), modeling a silly step in play or social gesture and

pausing expectantly, taking advantage of unexpected moments such as a tower of blocks about to fall by pausing and waiting for their initiation, and arranging toys in a nontransparent container or bag where the child pulls out items with different sensory textures and delights in their guesses as to what they discover as they share their enjoyment together with others (p. 223).

5) Lastly, to increase space for initiations from the child, the therapist should speak less. The practitioner should be mindful of how many words they are verbalizing and interjecting during their session time. It is okay to allow for moments of silence to increase spontaneous moments of meeting. Do not try and fill the space with words and questions to be productive. In addition, use more declaratives (statements) over imperatives (demanding questions) in your conversations to increase organic initiations.

6) A helpful strategy adapted from speech pathologists is to keep $MLU+1$ as a rule of thumb. MLU (or mean length of utterance) is the average number of words the child verbalizes independently in a sentence. Speech pathologists have their own specialized way of assessing this exact number. The practitioner can track the number of words heard in a child's sentence, over two or three visits, then calculate an average (such as two-word initiations, three-word initiations). Once we have ascertained a fair example, clinicians should respond in kind, while adding a bit extra for enrichment. An example is a child who typically speaks in four-word phrases on average (e.g. 'Let's feed the babydoll'). Here the clinician can track and respond with a four-word phrase + one extra enrichment word (e.g., 'Let's feed the babydoll milk'). And of course, be open to correction or acceptance of what we add to the play conversation.

7) The practitioner should also remember that the child may prefer to communicate nonverbally or they may use a device for communication. The practitioner can follow the same connection components in this intervention, regardless of the child's communication preferences.

Rationale

This non-directive play intervention does not have to be included in every session. It is most helpful in the beginning sessions of therapy, and then sprinkled in the middle sessions to help create space for shared joint attention, relationship-building initiations, consenting invitations to play, and opportunities for advancing communication. This is done with small but effective, targeted changes in the practitioner's environmental arrangement.

This play intervention helps develop improved connections with the practitioner and others. Comfortableness and confidence in increased initiations can lead to closer relationships with others, and to more confident ways to self-advocate one's needs, interests, thoughts, and ideas, without being dependent on the child's relationship partner to ask questions to them, direct their play, or take the lead. This play intervention can be taught to parents and caregivers who can practice and generalize initiation play during their special play time together. Children can gain the most benefit from this intervention if they practice this across settings, adults, friends, and their various play items of interest, as motivations may change over time.

References

Adamson, L.B., Bakeman, R., & Deckner, D.F. (2004). The development of symbol-infused joint engagement. *Child Development*, 75(4), 1171–1187.

Kasari, C., Gulsrud, A., Shire, S., & Strawbridge, C. (2022). *The JASPER Model for Children with Autism: Promoting Joint Attention, Symbolic Play, Engagement, and Regulation*. Guilford Press.

What Can You Do?

Therapy Needs: Advocacy
Level: Child, adolescent
Materials: Pictures of people in various situations or doing things. These can be cut out of magazines
Modality: Individual, family

Introduction

Neurodivergent children and adolescents may encounter environments and systems that are ableist and do not allow them to process and navigate in the way their system operates the best. In many cases, the child may be able to advocate for needs or processes and institute change. What Can You Do helps children conceptualize situations where someone may need to advocate and in what way(s) would they advocate.

Instructions

1) The practitioner should prepare this intervention before the session by cutting out several pictures of people in various situations or doing things that could provide examples of someone needing to advocate. The practitioner may need to begin with a general explanation of advocacy processes.

2) The practitioner shows a picture to the child or adolescent and asks them to think about what this person might need to advocate for and how they would advocate. The intervention can begin with silly thoughts such as 'He needs to go to McDonalds' and 'He can tell them his brain can't think until he has some chicken nuggets'. The practitioner can also participate and share an advocacy thought.

3) The idea is to help the child get used to what advocacy means and how it may be done.

4) The practitioner would then share another picture and repeat the process. As the intervention goes on, the responses could become more serious and more relevant to some of the child's situations.
5) Play continues until all the pictures have been discussed or the practitioner and child are no longer interested. This is an intervention that can be repeated in future sessions. Advocacy is a concept that will likely be an ongoing therapy goal to help the child understand and execute.

Rationale

Advocacy is an important ability for neurodivergent children and adolescents. This play intervention provides psychoeducation and exploration about how to advocate in a game format. It begins at a slower, more fun/engaging pace and progresses to a deeper understanding that children can apply to themselves. This intervention could be implemented as a family play session including the parents, who may also need to better understand advocacy work.

A Puppets Advocacy Story

Therapy Needs: Advocacy, social navigation
Level: Child
Materials: A variety of puppets
Modality: Individual, family

Introduction

Younger children may have a difficult time understanding advocacy and will need to begin learning about this concept at a level they can understand and implement. This play intervention utilizes puppets and a story-telling method to help neurodivergent children learn about advocating for their needs, preferences, and processes. The practitioner will need to supply two to four puppets that can be used in the intervention.

Instructions

1) The practitioner explains to the child that they are going to conduct a puppet show.
2) The show is going to be about a child who is at school, and something is making them feel uncomfortable. The practitioner will want to help direct this to something that the child is experiencing or something that is relevant to them. This might be a sensory sensitivity, a social navigation need, an anxiety-producing situation, a body autonomy issue, etc.
3) The child can pick out puppets for each character that will be in the story.

4) The practitioner and child create a story describing who are the characters, what is the issue, and how the main character will advocate for their need. The show should have a specific environment, a character who is uncomfortable with something that is happening or they are experiencing, a process where they advocate to another person their need, and a positive outcome. The practitioner will want the child to contribute as much as possible and remember to match the story and language to the child's level of understanding.
5) Once the story has been created, the practitioner and child perform the puppet show.
6) The practitioner and child can discuss how the main character advocated for themselves and how this might be important for the child to do sometime in their life.
7) Additional advocacy situation puppet shows can be created and played.

Rationale

This play intervention is designed for younger neurodivergent children to help them begin to understand the concept of advocacy. The practitioner should understand that this is a beginning to understanding advocacy and can consider ways for progressing the child's understanding and implementation. Parents can be involved in this intervention and continue to support advocacy understanding at home.

That Does Not Sound the Way it Looks

Therapy Needs: Social navigation, communication, advocacy
Level: Child, adolescent
Materials: None
Modality: Individual

Introduction

This play intervention is designed to help children and adolescents recognize their communication style and the confusing communication styles that others may exhibit. Further, it helps children and adolescents navigate more accurate understanding and meaning when observing and listening to others, and how to respond to someone who is presenting in a confusing manner.

Instructions

1) The practitioner tells the child that they are going to practice identifying situations when communicating with others and the interaction is not

making sense. The practitioner asks the child to say, draw, or write down how they most like to communicate to other people.

2) The practitioner and child discuss if the child's preferred ways of communicating change from one person to another, or from one type of situation to another. For example, is it different at home vs at school?

3) The practitioner also asks the child to say, draw, or write down different experiences they have had with other people where the other person was confusing for the child. For example, the way my English teacher talks or the way my grandfather looks at me.

4) The practitioner tells the child that they are going to try some different examples of situations that may be confusing and some situations where the child can communicate in the way they prefer. For example, the practitioner may say 'I am happy' in an angry voice with angry body language. The child can share what does not make sense about what the practitioner presented. For example, the child might say, 'Your face and the sound of your voice did not seem happy even though you said you were happy.' The practitioner can help the child communicate what is confusing in a way that the child prefers to communicate.

5) Some other examples the practitioner might give include saying, 'I am sad,' with a happy face and upbeat body language, or saying, 'I really like going to the park,' with a sad face and sad tone of voice. Examples could also include someone asking the child to look at their eyes while they are speaking to them or using slang, idioms, or even getting too close to them physically when talking to them.

6) The practitioner should have several examples prepared before the session with the child. The practitioner can also ask the child if they would like to create some examples.

7) The goal is to create discussion about how the child prefers to communicate and being able to address others who are being confusing.

8) Affirming note: This intervention is designed to empower the child to advocate for their ways of communicating and to address others who are being confusing or uncomfortable in the way they are trying to communicate with the child. Ideally, we would also want others who are interacting with child to be respectful of the way the child communicates and put forth the same efforts in the communication process as we are asking the neurodivergent child to do.

Rationale

Autistic and other neurodivergent children regularly have their preferred ways of communicating devalued and ignored. Neurotypical individuals often expect the neurodivergent child to interact with them in the way they believe is correct and make little effort to recognize or appreciate a different way of communicating. This play intervention helps children and adolescents work on understanding and appreciating the way they communicate. It also works on helping children recognize what is confusing and uncomfortable about how others communicate and how to address these situations. Parents can be taught how to implement this intervention and encouraged to play at home with their child.

I'm Going

Therapy Needs: Advocacy, social navigation	
Level: Child, adolescent	
Materials: Index cards	
Modality: Individual, family, group	

Introduction

Neurodivergent children and adolescents will typically need education and practice in regard to learning advocacy processes and skills. Advocacy can manifest in various ways and often it changes via the environment that someone is navigating. The I'm Going intervention helps children and adolescents identify possible advocacy needs in a particular environment and practice how they would advocate for themselves.

Instructions

1) The practitioner explains to the child that they are going to play a game identifying and practicing advocacy for certain environments. The practitioner may need to provide some basic information about the concept of advocacy.
2) The practitioner and child write various 'I'm going' environments on index cards. Some example environments include 'I'm going to school', 'I'm going to an amusement park', 'I'm going to a restaurant', 'I'm going to a friend's house', 'I'm going to church', and 'I'm going to the doctor's office' (a sample I'm Going card set is provided in the Appendix).
3) The index cards are placed face down in a pile and the practitioner and child take turns drawing the cards. When a card is drawn, both the practitioner and the child (the practitioner should go first) each talk about something that could be an advocacy need in that environment.
4) If the child were able, the practitioner and child could also talk about a way or how to advocate for a need in the environment. For example, the 'I am going to school card' is drawn and the child might say, 'I am going to school, and I don't want people to physically touch me.' The practitioner and child may also be able to add how to do this advocacy work by saying something like, 'I can have my parents tell the teacher or I can tell the teacher that it is physically painful for me.' This could be explored in many ways that would be specific to the child, such as draw a picture or write a note or send an email to advocate.

5) The practitioner should try to write eight to ten situations on index cards. The situations should be real situations that the child would participate in and may be having struggles with something that could need advocating.
6) Play continues until all the cards are completed. Parents can also be involved in this intervention as a family play therapy session.

Rationale

This play intervention helps children and adolescents in understanding about advocacy by examining several different environments and the possible advocacy needs in each environment. Advocacy is a process that develops over time and children will need practice to understand the concept and to implement it. This intervention (as with any advocacy intervention) may be best completed as a family intervention involving the parents. Often parents need to learn advocacy processes for their child and become the front-line person in helping their child learn how to advocate.

Home and School

Therapy Needs: Advocacy	
Level: Child, adolescent	
Materials: Paper, markers	
Modality: Individual	

Introduction

Children and adolescents are often navigating two primary environments – home and school. Often, these two environments hold the most potential for being misunderstood, not having needs met, and being devalued as a neurodivergent person. The Home and School intervention is designed to help children identify what is working well for them and what they may need in each of these environments (neurodivergent processes that are not being valued and needs not being met).

Instructions

1) The practitioner instructs the child to draw a picture of their school on one side of a piece of paper and a picture of their home on the other side of the paper.
2) The child is then instructed to choose a specific pen color and write all the things that they like, things that go well, ways they feel good, etc. on each picture for each environment.
3) The child is then instructed to choose a different pen color and write all the things they do not like, that do not feel good, that do not go well for them in each picture of each environment.

4) The practitioner and child then go through each environment and talk about what the child has written.
5) For things that are not going well, the practitioner and child can discuss ways to advocate for specific needs or issues. The advocating ideas can be written around the environment picture in a third color of pen.
6) It is often helpful to involve parents in this intervention as they will likely be a part of the child's advocacy. Many children, unless they are older teens, will require an adult to help them with advocacy efforts. If this intervention identifies a real advocacy need that should be addressed, the practitioner and/or parent will likely need to be involved to help with the advocacy efforts.

Rationale

The focus of this play intervention is on helping children and adolescents better understand, identify, and implement advocacy efforts. It is completed via a drawing activity which may be a play presence for some children and help them better understand the concept. Parents can be a part of this intervention. They may need to address issues with the school and help their child advocate. Also the practitioner and parents may need to meet and discuss home needs that require advocacy change for the child.

Advocacy Collage

Therapy Needs: Advocacy, identity
Level: Child, adolescent
Materials: Medium to large piece of card stock or paper, magazines, scissors, glue
Modality: Individual, group

Introduction

Understanding advocacy efforts can almost be considered synonymous with being neurodivergent. Often children and adolescents do not know what advocacy means or how they would begin to implement advocacy processes. This play intervention creates a strong visual representation of understanding advocacy. The collage creation may be especially appealing for children who have art and creative expression play preferences.

Instructions

1) The practitioner explains to the child that they will be creating a collage.
2) The practitioner should have the collage materials present and ready to use.
3) The practitioner will explain that the collage is going to be about the concept of advocacy. The practitioner may need to explain advocacy to the child and the explanation should be age-appropriate.

4) The practitioner will then ask the child to look through the magazines and cut out anything they find that can be used in the collage to remind them of advocacy or that explains advocacy. The practitioner can help cut out things as well. The practitioner will want to make sure key components of advocacy are represented.
5) Once things have been cut out from the magazines, the collage is assembled on some type of large white paper. A card stock material is usually better for creating the collage.
6) Once the collage has been created, the practitioner and child can go through the whole collage, talking about each component of advocacy.
7) The child can take the collage home to reference and remind them of advocacy awareness.

Rationale

This play intervention uses expressive play to help children learn about advocacy. It is important for neurodivergent children to learn about advocacy and to understand how advocacy can be implemented. This intervention also helps children better understand and value their own identity and how to advocate for their needs.

I Can Use My Voice

Therapy Needs: Advocacy
Level: Child, adolescent
Materials: Toy or real microphone
Modality: Individual, group

Introduction

This play game intervention focuses on the child practicing telling someone how they feel, that they do not like something, and that they need something. It is implemented in a playful atmosphere, allowing the child to explore different advocacy situations and feel more confident in advocating for their needs.

Instructions

1) The practitioner provides a toy or real microphone for the child.
2) The practitioner explains they are going to practice and/or role-play advocating for themselves.
3) The practitioner and child create a few scenarios where the child may need to advocate. The practitioner may need to explain the concept of

advocacy and provide some examples. The child can think of scenarios, but the practitioner will likely need to assist.

4) Once the scenarios have been established. The child uses the microphone and practices standing up and advocating. This may be asking for help from a teacher, or telling a child they do not like what they are doing, or telling an adult that something is bothering their senses. Advocacy does not have to be verbal. Other methods of communicating advocacy can also be explored and practiced.

5) As the child displays advocacy, the practitioner should respond with encouragement to the child. The practitioner and child can continue this intervention until they have practiced all their scenarios.

Rationale

This play intervention is designed to help children learn about and practice advocacy efforts. Different scenarios can be created to practice, and the scenarios should be applicable to the child's life. This intervention can be repeated in multiple sessions to help the child gain awareness and confidence in advocating for themselves.

Help Me

Therapy Needs: Advocacy	
Level: Child	
Materials: Puppets or miniatures	
Modality: Individual	

Introduction

This play intervention helps children conceptualize advocacy situations and how to advocate for needs. The intervention is done in a creative story process using puppets or miniatures. The practitioner and child create a story that allows the characters to experience advocating for needs.

Instructions

1) The practitioner explains to the child that they are going to create a story using puppets (miniatures can also be used in place of puppets).

2) The story will be about someone (a puppet) who is experiencing a situation that is a problem for them, such as another person being mean to them, or the light in the room hurting their eyes. This is something they need help with. Another person (puppet) helps them figure out how to advocate for themselves in order to solve their problem.

3) The practitioner and child then create the puppet story they are going to perform. The practitioner should encourage the child to create as much of the story as they can. The practitioner can interject and add as needed to keep the advocacy focus.
4) Once the story has been created, the practitioner and child perform the puppet story. The practitioner can process the story with the child, asking them about situations in their own life that may need advocacy.
5) The practitioner and child can create more puppet stories and continue the play if the child is interested.

Rationale

Neurodivergent children often are in situations that require advocacy. Adults can advocate for children, but it is empowering for children to learn about advocacy and how to advocate for themselves. This play intervention provides the opportunity to learn about advocacy through metaphor-based play.

Stepping Tiles Advocacy

Therapy Needs: Advocacy, sensory needs
Level: Child, adolescent
Materials: Five to six stepping tiles
Modality: Individual

Introduction

Some neurodivergent children with sensory needs enjoy the process of stepping on various types of play stepping tiles. These can be rubber, squishy, colorful, any type of texture or substance. This intervention pairs this sensory activity with learning about and practicing advocacy.

Instructions

1) The practitioner displays five to six stepping tiles and has the child place them around the room.
2) The practitioner explains that the child is going to step, hop, or jump from one stone to the other until they have gotten through all of them.
3) As the child lands on a stone, they will practice an advocacy statement. The practitioner and child can discuss real scenarios where the child may need to advocate for themselves.
4) The practitioner and child will write down what type of advocacy statement will be done for each stone.
5) The child is now ready to begin their journal. They will move in whatever way has been established to the first stone and make their first advocacy

statement. They will then go to the second stone and make their next advocacy statement. This continues until they have gotten through all the stones.

6) The intervention can be repeated with the same advocacy statement for more practice or repeated with new statements.

7) Play can continue until the child is no longer interested.

Rationale

This play intervention combines sensory-related needs with advocacy needs. Sensory tiles are used in the game play as children practice advocacy statements. Ideally, the play intervention can be implemented multiple times in different sessions. Children will likely need repeated practice to understand advocacy implementation.

Appendix

Note: For those who have purchased the book, copies of inventories and worksheets found in the Appendix can be accessed in PDF version on the AutPlay Therapy website in the protected area on the Resources page. Contact the AutPlay Therapy Clinic for a passcode.

Feelings List

Accepted	Afraid	Affectionate	Loyal
Angry	Miserable	Anxious	Misunderstood
Peaceful	Beautiful	Playful	Ashamed
Brave	Awkward	Calm	Proud
Capable	Quiet	Bored	Overwhelmed
Caring	Relaxed	Confused	Cheerful
Relieved	Defeated	Comfortable	Safe
Competent	Satisfied	Concerned	Mad
Depressed	Pressured	Confident	Provoked
Content	Desperate	Regretful	Courageous
Silly	Lonely	Rejected	Curious
Special	Disappointed	Remorseful	Strong
Discouraged	Disgusted	Sad	Sympathetic
Excited	Embarrassed	Shy	Forgiving
Thankful	Sorry	Friendly	Thrilled
Fearful	Stubborn	Nervous	Stupid
Glad	Understood	Frustrated	Good
Unique	Furious	Tired	Grateful
Valuable	Guilty	Touchy	Great
Hateful	Happy	Helpless	Hopeful
Wonderful	Hopeless	Humorous	Worthwhile
Unattractive	Joyful	Uncertain	Lovable
Humiliated	Uncomfortable	Loved	Hurt
Ignored	Impatient	Indecisive	Inferior
Insecure	Irritated	Jealous	Worried

Toys and Materials List

Functional Toys
Kitchen • Food • Dishes • Baby Dolls • Doll house • Miniature People Miniature
Animals • Cars, Trucks, Boats • Bowling Set
Basketball Goal • Cash Register • Doctor's Kit • Tool Kit
Ring Toss • Dart Board • Toy Phone • Toy Camera • Toy Phone
Hairdresser Kit • Dentist Kit

Expressive and Constructive Materials
Paper • Markers and Crayons • Paints • Playdough • Putty
Clay • Dry Erase Board and Markers • Stickers • Beads
Ribbon • Pipe Cleaners • Confetti • Pom Poms • Train Track • Race Track
Puppets • Dress-Up Clothes and Hats • Mr. Potato Head • LEGO® • Blocks

Sensory Toys
Sand Tray • Water Tray • Moon Sand • Kinetic Sand
Rice or Bean Tray • Snow Mobility • Sensory Balls
Theraputty • Tangle Toys • Sidewalk Chalk • Fidget Toys
Musical Instruments • Slinky • Whirly Wheel • Koosh Ball • Magnets Punching
BagHoola Hoops • Bean Bags • Brain Puzzles • Light-Up Objects
Balloons • Bubbles • Ring Toss • Rubik's Cube • Origami Kit
Mini Trampoline • Word Search • Word Scramble • Seek and Find Games

Boardgames
Find It • Bop It • Jenga • Chairs • Pick-Up Sticks
Jacks • Barrel of Monkeys • Animal Logic
Blokus • Rush Hour • Twister • Spot It • Stare
I Spy • Story Cubes • Memory • Chicky Boom • HedBanz
Sorry • Trouble • Forbidden Island • Secret Door

Digital Toys
iPad or Tablet • Nintendo Switch • VR • Game Console • Computer
Smart Phone • Smart TV

Play-Based Intervention Tracking Sheet

PlayIntervention	Need Area Addressed (emotional, social, connection, advocacy, sensory, self-worth, regulation, etc.)	Date Administered	Child/Adolescent Response

Create Your Own Intervention Worksheet

Name of Intervention:_____

Area(s) Addressed (circle all that apply): Feeling Identification, Regulation, Social, Connection, Advocacy, Other:_____

Level (circle one): Child, Adolescent
Modality (circle all that apply): Individual, Family, Group

Materials Needed:

_____
_____
_____
_____
_____

Practitioners should be able to answer the following questions with a yes response:

Is this a structured play intervention?

Is the play considered the agent of change?

Does the intervention address needs the child is struggling with?

Does the intervention align with the child's therapy goals?

Can the intervention be adjusted from simple to more complex?

Is the intervention low prop?

Is the intervention simple to explain and complete (not too many steps)?

Can the practitioner participate with and assist the child if needed?

Can the intervention be taught to parents to implement at home?

Is the intervention free of ableist constructs and affirming for the child?

Description of Intervention Including Theoretical Underpinnings:

_____
_____
_____
_____

_____
_____
_____
_____
_____
_____
_____
_____
_____
_____
_____
_____

Goals of Intervention:

_____
_____
_____
_____
_____
_____
_____
_____
_____
_____
_____
_____
_____
_____

Additional Information:

_____
_____
_____
_____
_____
_____
_____
_____
_____
_____
_____
_____
_____
_____
_____
_____

AutPlay Therapy Assessment of Play Inventory (modified)

Child's Name_____Age_____Gender_____Date_____

Read the following play categories and definitions, and rate where you feel the child is at in terms of possessing and demonstrating this type of play.

Functional Play is a term also used for relational play; it means denoting use of objects in play for the purposes for which they were intended, e.g., using simple objects correctly, combining related objects, and making objects do what they are made to do (setting up a bowling set and bowling).

NO – 12345678910 – YES

Symbolic Play refers to symbolic, or pretend play, which occurs when children begin to substitute one object for another. For example, using a hairbrush to represent a microphone. The child may pretend to do something (with or without the object present or with an object representing another object) or be someone.

NO – 12345678910 – YES

Cooperative Play refers to a play where children plan, assign roles, and play together. Cooperative play is goal-oriented and children play in an organized manner toward a common end. Moreover, cooperative play is a 'true social play' in which children cooperate or assume reciprocal roles.

NO – 12345678910 – YES

Sociodramatic Play refers to play involving acting out scripts, scenes, and plays adapted from cartoons, books. Children take/assume roles using themselves and/or characters like dolls and puppets as they interact together on common themes.

NO – 12345678910 – YES

Peer Play refers to interactions with one's peers, which provide opportunities for physical, cognitive, social, and emotional development.

NO – 12345678910 – YES

Constructive Play is characterized as manipulation of objects for the purpose of constructing or creating something. Children use materials to achieve a specific goal in mind that requires transformation of objects into a new configuration. LEGO® pieces turned into cars or houses are an example of this play.

NO – 12345678910 – YES

Sensory Play involves playing with toys or items for the purpose of sensory sensations or sensory seeking. Enjoying the toy or object because of how it feels or what it produces for the senses. Sensory balls, putty, and swings are examples.

NO – 12345678910 – YES

Technology Play is characterized by playing online and video games alone or with others. This might involve a tablet, a game station, a VR system, smartphone, or playing games on a computer.

NO – 12345678910 – YES

AutPlay Therapy Assessment of Play Inventory (modified)

Child's Name_____Age_____Gender_____Date_____

Please answer the following questions regarding the child's play. Try to think about specific times you have observed or played with the child and answer the questions as completely as possible.

Does the child play with toys?

Does the child play independently?

Does the child initiate play?

Does the child interact during play?

What type of play does the child seem to like?

What types of toys or materials does the child seem drawn toward?

If you ask the child to play, what does the child do?

Does the child seem to want to play?

Does the child seem to like technology-based play?

Describe the child's play.

Friend Mapping Worksheet

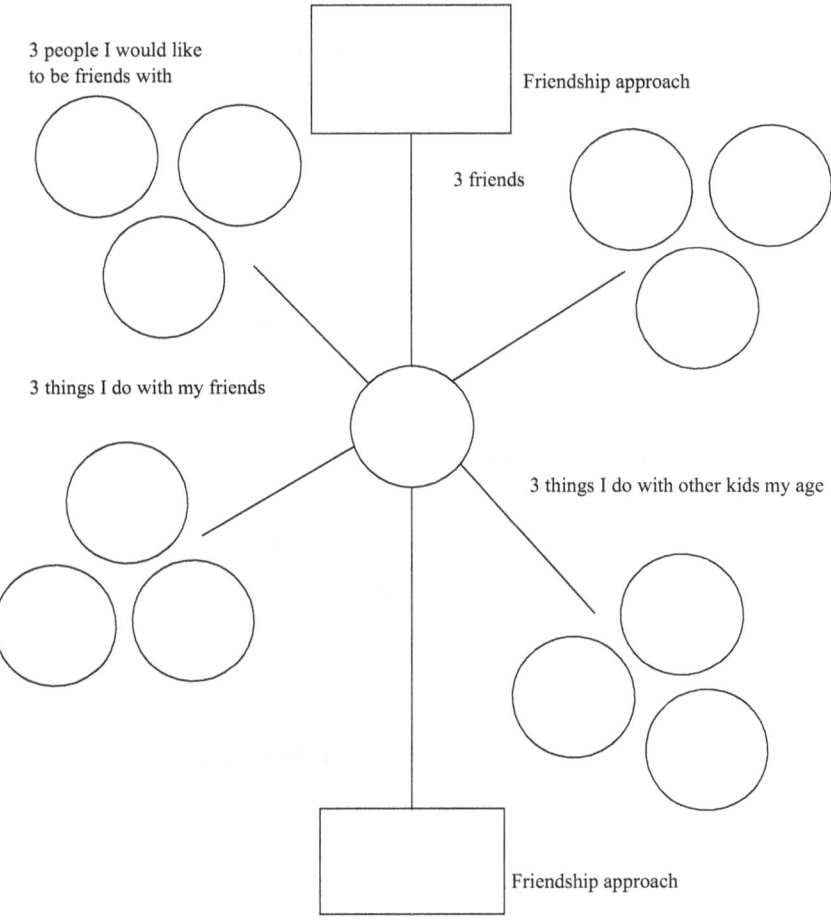

Figure A.1 Friend mapping worksheet.

Feelings Pick-Up Sticks Feelings/Color Sheet

RED Happy • Confused • Scared • Proud • Annoyed
BLUE Sad • Worried • Loved • Excited • Upset
GREEN Angry • Calm • Nervous • Silly • Energized
YELLOW Brave • Frustrated • Tired • Friendly • Bored
BLACK Peaceful • Anxious • Normal

Write a Feelings Story Templates

_____ happy _____
_____ sad _____
_____ shy _____
loved _____
_____ angry _____
_____ excited _____ worried _____
_____

_____ happy _____
_____ sad _____
_____ shy _____
loved _____
_____ angry _____

_____ excited _____ worried _____
_____

_____ happy _____
_____ sad _____
_____ shy _____
loved _____
_____ angry _____
_____ excited _____ worried _____
_____

Feeling List Stop Worksheet

1) _____

2) _____

3) _____

4) _____

5) _____

6) _____

7) _____

8) _____

9) _____

10) _____

11) _____

12) _____

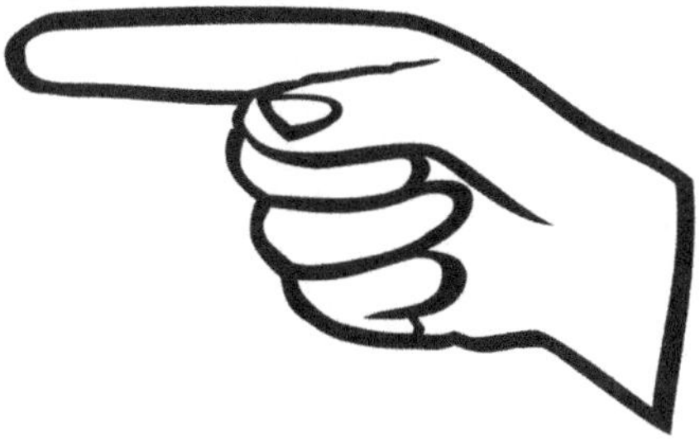

Figure A.2

I Sense Story Worksheet

Child's Name_____

Name of Story_____

Looks Like

_____

Sounds Like

_____

Smells Like

_____

Tastes Like

_____

Feels Like

_____

Moves Like

_____

I Can Do That Game

Action Cards

Hop Across the Room	Walk Backwards	Hop in One Place	Walk Around the Room	Skip in a Circle
Crawl	Jump Three Times	Run in Place	Dance	Act Silly

Object Cards

With a Ball	With a Stuffed Animal	With a Hat	With a Pillow	With a Doll
With a Toy	With a Piece of Paper	With a Hula Hoop	With a Bean Bag	With a Plate

Body Part Cards

Between your Knees	On your Head	At your Feet	On your Back	Under your Right Arm
Under your Arm	In your Left Hand	Under Both Arms	Under your Chin	In your Right Hand

I'm Going Card Set

I'm going to school	I'm going to a restaurant	I'm going to the doctor's office
I'm going to get my hair cut	I'm going to a friend's house	I'm going to church
I'm going to the grocery store	I'm going for a ride in the car	I'm going to a party
I'm going to the dentist office	I'm going to the shoe store	I'm going to a park
I'm going to the mall	I'm going for a walk	I'm going to the post office
I'm going to the dentist	I'm going to my grandparents' house	I'm going to an amusement park

Index